Open your Heart with
Kundalini Yoga

Siri Datta

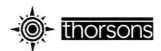

Thorsons
An Imprint of HarperCollins*Publishers*
77–85 Fulham Palace Road
Hammersmith, London W6 8JB

The website address is:
www.thorsonselement.com

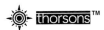 ™

and *Thorsons* are trademarks of
HarperCollins*Publishers* Limited

First published by Thorsons 2003

1 3 5 7 9 10 8 6 4 2

© Siri Datta, 2003

Siri Datta asserts the moral right to
be identified as the author of this work

A catalogue record of this book
is available from the British Library

ISBN 0 00 714680 9

Photographs © Guy Hearn
Text illustrations on pp. 2, 28, 34, 116, 170, 184 and 202 © Jane Spencer

Printed and bound in Great Britain by
Scotprint, Haddington, East Lothian

Contents

Acknowledgements

To all the Souls who pick up this book;

to Yogi Bhajan, who came to the West with the teachings of Kundalini Yoga;

to my beloved parents, Dinah and Patrick Cuddihy;

to Darryl O'Keeffe and Guru Dharam Singh, who taught me this sacred science;

to Susanna Abbott and Victoria McCulloch, who believed in the cause;

to Alan Cunliffe; who made sense of it all;

to the Virtual Circle;

to Anrul Ullah, the embodiment of love;

to the Christ Consciousness that has filled my Soul since the practice reminded me who, I AM;

to my courageous and brilliant best friends, Sidonie Barton, Rebecca Hutley, Emma Field-Rayner and James Fenner;

and to Paul Goodwin, who I have known and loved forever...

You are all, but One.

Welcome

There has always been a hidden pathway, a secret technology, to activate our full potential, and a mystical password that can wake up humanity. The original blueprint is wrapped away inside each one of us and the technology to unleash that abundance is Kundalini Yoga.

This book is a step-by-step guide on how to practise Kundalini Yoga and meditation. Full of advice on how to handle modern-day stress and tension, simple and easy techniques that anyone can do to beat addictions, depression and to balance the mind and emotions. Kundalini Yoga works from the inside out. All layers of our being will fall back into alignment as we work through the practice.

This yoga is the all-encompassing system to balance the pace and challenges of twenty-first-century life.

In my humble opinion this book is greatly needed now for humanity and the present stage of evolution of the Universe. We will require tools and understanding as we move at a rapid pace towards the vibration of the heart. As we shred layers of illusion and negativity, so we will step into our true essence and embody pure love, pure joy and pure truth.

Siri Datta

Caution

Kundalini Yoga, like all forms of yoga, involves using your muscles, tendons, ligaments, joints and mind in novel and unfamiliar ways. While all the movements are possible, and none of them is inherently harmful, you must be careful. Many of the movements are so different from those that you are used to that you must approach them patiently and gradually. Do not rush, do not push, and do not force your body. While you may get away with it sometimes, there are some parts of the body, where you may not. Muscles, once strained, will repair: tendons and ligaments may not. The knees and the neck are especially vulnerable.

Kundalini Yoga is not simply a form of exercise. It is an extremely potent form of transformation. The postures, bandhs and the breathing, even when done partially or with difficulty, bring about great changes in your energetic equilibrium. This can precipitate the release of deep psychic blocks. If they are not consciously met and allowed to resolve themselves, they can have a disturbing effect on the mind and body. Pay attention to your actions at all times, feeling their effects, and responding accordingly.

When you are carrying out the breathing exercises be aware that if you feel dizzy or faint, stop immediately. Pranayama, the yogic breathing technique, is the most powerful way to alter consciousness, and should be treated with the utmost respect.

As a student of Kundalini Yoga you should let your teacher know if you are being treated for any medical condition, and especially if you are taking any prescribed drugs. If you are suffering from an illness or injury, please consult a medical professional and an experienced, trained yoga teacher before using this book. The therapeutic aspect of Kundalini Yoga is one that should not be taken for granted. In order to use its specific therapeutic purposes, you should find a teacher who is fully trained and experienced in that application. At the back of this book (see page 231) there is a list of contacts to find teachers world wide.

Under no circumstances should you practise Kundalini Yoga while under the influence of any controlled substances (drugs or alcohol).

Practical considerations

- Yoga is most beneficial if you practise it regularly. A daily practice of 20 minutes is good. Otherwise two to three times per week will produce obvious results.
- Morning practice sets you up for the day; whereas evening practice will find you more flexible. Both times have disadvantages and advantages.
- Practise on a natural mat; cotton or wool is best. Sheepskins have been a traditional choice since ancient times.
- Never force or push yourself physically in a posture.
- Never practise in a draught, although the room should be well ventilated.
- Practise in a warm room, as your muscles are being heated from within. Cold currents of air can weaken your practice.
- Practise at the same time, in the same place, if possible.
- Wear natural, loose clothing – preferably white – to expand the aura.
- If you are pregnant, tell your teacher, as there are postures and breathing exercises that you should not do.
- If you are injured or recovering from an injury, be patient and sensible.
- Practise on an empty stomach, bowels and bladder.
- Do not wipe sweat away; allow it to soak back into your skin naturally.
- If you suffer from high blood pressure or heart complaints tell your teacher, as there are postures and breathing exercises that you should not do.
- Tell your teacher about *all* your medical conditions, as well as prescribed and non-prescribed medication you may be taking.
- If you are experiencing the heaviest days of your period tell your teacher, as some breathing exercises and postures are not advised.
- When you need to, stop, but maintain the awareness and breathing, returning to the posture when you are ready to.
- When returning to practice after illness, go slowly and gently.
- Do not practise if you have consumed drugs or alcohol.
- If you have back complaints, tell your teacher, who will advise you of variations.
- Remember that yoga is union, not battle.

Foreword

We are changing. 'We' being the entire globe and all of humanity. We are finally leaving the adolescent stage of our development as conscious human beings and entering a new time, a new age, the Aquarian age – the age of experience, the age of knowledge. A shift in age is like a great tide. It raises all boats. Whether you do something or not, the tide rises. The shift we are going through reaches a full beginning by November 11, 2011. With it we will go through a fundamental change in how we relate to ourselves, each other and to the world. It is a change in consciousness. It is not just a change: it is a belief. It is change in how we hold beliefs and how we become believable in our beliefs and our deepest spiritual identity as human beings.

At the change of an age, by God's grace, many people, saints and guides emerge to help. Among those there will be a master of the consciousness of the age. And there will be tools with which we can elevate ourselves and match up to the progression and demands of the awakening age. Yogi Bhajan came to the west in 1969 and spoke as a Master and guide for the Aquarian Age. He started with a declaration, 'I have come to create teachers to serve the Aquarian Age, not to collect students'. He began to teach Kundalini Yoga.

Kundalini Yoga was recognized as the premier yoga to awaken the consciousness and potential of the individual. 'Kundalini' means awareness. Awareness is a property of the soul, of you, of your core existence. The awareness a raised kundalini gives you is not a product of the brain. It is a synchronization of your core being with the expression of that being using the full potential of your glandular and nervous systems. When kundalini is awakened you are aware of the impact of each word you speak. You sense the impact of your action before you take it. You do not try to control others or control the outcomes of things. You control the beginning. The beginning of the thought. The start of the journey. You live perpetual values: character, caliber, grace, compassion, fearlessness, service and generosity. These values arise not out of belief in their goodness or utility but out of the experience of who we are and how we are part of the Creator and Creation. Just as the fragrance of a rose is released automatically with its bloom, values are the fragrances of our spiritual blooming.

Kundalini Yoga was shrouded in myth and secrecy for centuries. Its power and potential was closely guarded in oral traditions and the qualifications to practise it were higher than going to a graduate school. You had to practise over two decades of Hatha Yoga, Mantra Yoga, pranayama and selfless service before you would be tested to qualify to learn a single kundalini kriya, a formula and discipline to awaken the Self. Sometimes it was taught to healers, rulers and families who had to show great character over generations.

In 1969 Yogi Bhajan broke the formula of the old age, the Piscean. He came as a postman. He delivered the legacy of humanity to excel and serve in this new time. He introduced the healing energy of Guru Ram Das. He taught to all without condition. For more than three decades he taught thousands of meditations and kriyas and laid the concept of how to live in the Aquarian Age.

This book carries on that tradition and brings it in a very accessible form to our contemporary culture. Siri Datta speaks in a friendly and enthusiastic voice that comes from practice and personal transformation. When you read this book and practise the teachings in it you may find an odd feeling of comfort arising from within. It is not something new; it is remembering who you are and gaining a discipline to act on that with integrity and excellence. As director of training in Kundalini Yoga for the Kundalini Research Institute I am grateful to Siri Datta for this enlightening and entertaining volume. I am infinitely grateful to all the work and blessings we have received from Yogi Bhajan and for his relentless efforts that have led to all the teachers serving, sharing and uplifting us all.

May you live healthy, happy and holy.
In the Naam,
Gurucharan Singh Khalsa, Ph.D.,
Director of Training KRI
www.Breathwalk.com

How to use this book

This book is an introductory guide to the practice of Kundalini Yoga. There are 21 sets and ten meditations, which will build a strong foundation for the understanding and experience of this sacred technology. There is also a section called Ancient Answers for Modern Living (*see page* 185), which gives a yogic exercise to help combat particular issues in your life ranging from Addiction to Depression.

The book has been divided into six parts. Part 1 (*see page* 3) covers the Introduction to Kundalini Yoga; what it is all about and where it came from. Part 2 (*see page* 35) goes into detail about the Science of Kundalini Yoga, how it works and the different layers that go into the practice, making it so quick to achieve transformation and awareness.

Part 3 (*see page* 117) contains the yoga sets. This part is divided into the three levels of our being: the body, the mind and the soul. You can choose any set at any time, depending on how you are feeling. You may decide you need a challenging physical set for the body, or you may decide you need something subtler, to work on your emotions.

Each section on the yoga sets has the following parts:

o   Detailed text and illustrations outlining the relevance of the exercise; what each posture involves; how long you should spend doing it; and sometimes a designated mantra.
o   Detailed instructions on the breathing pattern and the focus of your awareness.
o   A quote from either Yogi Bhajan or myself with the essence behind the set.

How long the sequence takes is up to you. Times have been specified, but during the initial stages of practice you can decrease the times. Take your time. Stay with a set until you know it by heart. A set will bring you greater benefits if you commit to practise it daily for 40 continuous days.

Part 4 (*see page* 171), covers four powerful but simple kundalini meditations, ideal for everyday practise. Part 5 (*see page* 185) is called Ancient Answers for Modern Living, while Part 6 (*see page* 203) completes the book with a chapter on the yogic lifestyle, diet, foods that heal and beauty advice. This final section is relevant to all forms of spiritual practice, as awareness of what we consume is of the utmost importance for strengthening the body and mind.

Please read the first part of the book before you begin the physical practice, as there are many facets of kundalini that you need to know about, making the practice complete. There is a sacred technology inherent within Kundalini Yoga and this gift is priceless. The only way to know this is to experience it for yourself. Kundalini Yoga works from the inside out, and it brings forth the key to transformation. Always follow the sets exactly as they are laid out in this book. In this way you can be sure that you are using a tried-and-tested method of achieving a powerful form of enlightenment.

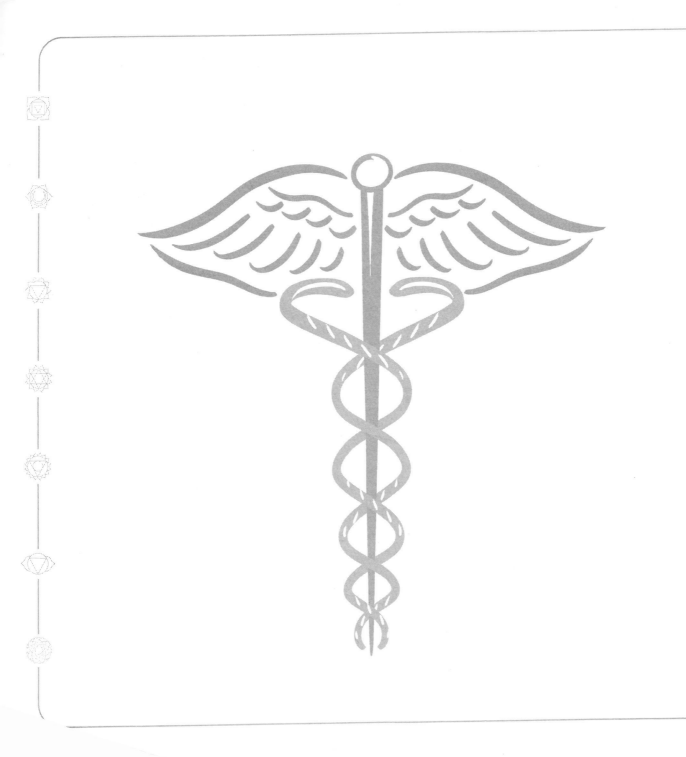

part one

An introduction
to Kundalini Yoga

What is Yoga?

Yoga is a complete science of life that originated in India many thousands of years ago. It is the oldest system of personal development in the world, encompassing the three-fold structure of humankind: the body, mind and spirit. The ancient yogis had a profound understanding of humankind's essential nature and what we need in order to live in harmony with our environment and ourselves. They perceived the body as the vehicle, the mind as the driver and the soul as humankind's true identity. Action, emotion and intelligence are the three forces that pull the body–vehicle. To achieve harmony these three forces must be in balance. The Kundalini Yoga system delivers this balance, leading to a sense of tremendous well-being.

Yoga is much needed in life because people have the right to know who they are and what it means to be a human being. The meaning of yoga in the West is radically different from that in the East. In the West it usually means the analytical study of knowledge and understanding, using the intellect. It is far removed from the experience and application of this knowledge. In the East, the understanding is kept to a minimum before the experience has been achieved. The driving force is to experience and apply the techniques, to take the action rather than try to understand how it works. For those in the West, this is a great disadvantage. Generally speaking, Westerners seem shy of physical commitment and discipline. But this is the test; life cannot be received unless it is given, too.

Anyone can practise yoga; all you need is a modest space and a strong desire to live a healthier, more fulfilled, life. Do not compare your own efforts with the illustrations of the more advanced yoga postures. Just start at the beginning and do what feels right for you. You are about to set off on an adventure in consciousness. Your only goal is the closing down of the outside world and the creation of a relationship with yourself. The word *yoga* literally means 'union', to merge. This is the merging of all three parts of yourself into one harmonious unit, or the greater meaning, which is to merge the finite with the infinite.

Yoga in your Life

People come to yoga for many reasons. They may want to keep fit and healthy, relieve stress, or perhaps they may want it to help with a specific complaint such as backache. Some people are attracted because they are searching for more meaning in their lives and they wish to find a greater understanding of themselves. Whatever the reason, yoga is a tool you can use to achieve what you want, and much more besides. At first glance yoga may resemble a series of stretches, breathing techniques and relaxation. But in time anyone who practises yoga will discover the real jewel that is often hidden during the initial stages. That jewel is the glimpse of your true nature, which is pure love and inner peace. This is the journey that we are all, consciously or unconsciously, gradually moving towards. There is no limit to what you can do – since only our illusions and preconceptions hold us back and prevent us from finding our true fulfilment.

The Physiology of Yoga

Just as we expect a car to depreciate in value with age, so we resign ourselves to the fact that as we get older, the body functions less efficiently with the passing years. This is another illusion. Ageing is largely an artificial condition, caused mainly by 'self-poisoning'. Through keeping the body parts 'clean' by practising yoga we can significantly reduce the catabolic process of cell deterioration.

In recent years the medical profession has started to look more closely at the effects of yoga. There have been cases in which conditions such as high blood pressure, chronic fatigue syndrome, asthma, heart conditions and varicose veins are effectively relieved through the practice of yoga. Laboratory tests have also confirmed that yogis have control over autonomic or involuntary functions such as body temperature, heartbeat and blood pressure. One study noted that over a six-month period of practising yoga the following effects were recorded: significantly increased lung capacity; reduced body weight; improved ability to resist stress; and a decrease in cholesterol and blood sugar levels. According to ancient yogic tradition it is understood that with regular practice you can calm your mind, strengthen your body and allow your soul to shine through. Today there can no longer be any doubt about yoga's effectiveness as both a curative and preventative medicine.

The History of Yoga

The origins of yoga are shrouded in the mists of time – for yoga is regarded as a Divine science of life, revealed to enlightened sages while they are in the depths of meditation. Yoga is not a religion. When you break the word 'religion' down you will reach a greater understanding of the word, which is 'realized origin'. Our origin is undoubtedly that of spirit and pure love.

According to the ancient scriptures there is evidence of yoga in the *Rigveda* (Knowledge of Praise), dating from 5,000 BC. It is clearly in use and acknowledged as an ancient practice in the B*hagavadgita* (Lord's Song), 2,500 BC.

The Meaning of Yoga

The word *yoga* originates from the Sanskrit root word jugit, which literally means 'union'. In the West it is known to come from the biblical word 'yoke', which translates into the understanding 'to join together'. The underlying purpose of all forms of yoga is to reunite all three aspects of ourselves, to join with the Infinite Self. Union with this Infinite Self (God) or 'pure consciousness' liberates the spirit from all sense of separation, freeing it from the illusion of death. Even in our ignorance the human spirit often perceives that something is lacking in life, something that neither achieving a goal nor fulfilling a desire can truly satisfy.

What is Kundalini Yoga?

Throughout the ages, in every civilization, there has been a hidden pathway, a secret technology of discovery, which enables the individual to reach the ultimate potential. This is a technique that has the ability to elevate, inspire and awaken the individual to their own greatness. That greatness is within every one of us, and the technology that can do this is Kundalini Yoga.

As an enthusiastic teacher of Kundalini Yoga, I am always asked 'What is it? Is it like Hatha Yoga, or Ashtanga Yoga? Is it dynamic or static? Are there meditation or breathing techniques?' My answer is always the same: it is all of those things, and a multitude more.

Yogi Bhajan, the Master of Kundalini Yoga, now living in New Mexico, has explained that there are 22 major forms of yoga, each one expressing a facet of the whole. A good way of understanding this is that each different form of yoga is like the facet of a diamond. The diamond herself is Kundalini Yoga, the mother of all yogas.

Kundalini Yoga is the most inclusive of all yoga practices as it includes all aspects of yoga within its teachings. In this practice there are over 8.4 million kriyas (completed sequences, or sets). These kriyas are made up of asanas (postures), pranayama (breathing exercises), mantra (chanting), mudras (hand gestures), bandhs (body locks) and meditation.

The kriyas are a blend of dynamic and static postures that deliver a perfect sequence of energy, tones and feelings played upon the instrument of the body. In the ancient scriptures it is said that Kundalini Yoga is the fastest way to create the transformation that the individual is seeking. There is a certain depth, completeness and timelessness that is inherent in Kundalini Yoga.

Kundalini Yoga is a legacy. It has been practised as an exact science by masters in communication with Infinity, coming directly from the Soul. It is a practice that has been experienced and handed down through enlightened souls for many thousands of years. It is said that Christ, Buddha and Moses practised Kundalini Yoga.

In ancient times it was often taught and passed down through the line of kings. These Kundalini Yoga masters did not specifically or personally pass on the knowledge. Rather it is thought that the teachings were handed down via an authentic lineage of Raj (Royal) Yogis. Kundalini Yoga knowledge was transmitted through meditation and altered states. It was this practice that was kept within the bloodline of royalty. We understand that the very first transmission of Kundalini Yoga was passed to the Hindu god Shiva, who in turn passed the knowledge to his consort Parvarti. From the B*hagavadgita* we can understand that Lord Krishna was a keeper of the teachings, which were then passed to King Janaka, who was an early Raj Yogi and master of Kundalini Yoga. This was passed on through that lineage to Guru Ram Das, a Guru of the Sikhs, via the subtle realms. Guru Ram Das was bestowed the High Throne of Raj Yoga, known as the Takhat. The word *takhat* literally means 'high throne' and is not specific to any exclusive form of yoga; there are many other takhats. This meant that he had to pass the technology on with his blessing to anyone who came along. It was through Guru Ram Das that the teachings were passed on to Yogi Bhajan. In 1969 Yogi Bhajan took Kundalini Yoga to the United States, against the wishes of his peers. Until then, it had always been highly secret and was never practised in public.

Since Kundalini Yoga has become so popular in the United States the Kundalini Research Institute (KRI) has been developed. This was founded to verify, promote, produce and preserve the teachings of Yogi Bhajan, exactly as they had been passed down.

There is much confusion surrounding kundalini and Kundalini Yoga. Some experts say that it is the most potent and powerful way to change consciousness, while others warn against practising it, or veil the entire teaching in secrecy. Yet how can something as essential to consciousness as kundalini be feared? Some people worry about raising the kundalini energy, but teachings from Yogi Bhajan have dispelled many misrepresentations and myths surrounding kundalini and his explicit teachings have given researchers techniques that can be thoroughly tested out.

Kundalini Yoga is also known as the 'yoga of awareness'. Awareness leads to understanding and understanding gives way to acceptance. When you can accept yourself, all your limitations fade away. All your fears, insecurities, and self-belittlement cease to be. In its place are abundance, hope and the wisdom of your true worth. Kundalini Yoga is so much more than a set of physical exercises. If genuinely practised, with respect and reverence, it will change your life.

There is only one way that you can practise Kundalini Yoga. It is very specific, clearly laid out and it is practised as it was given, with no alterations. Its path can take you to many places, whether you wish to achieve enlightenment or to release parts of yourself that are out of date and do not reflect the person you wish to be. Kundalini Yoga can also offer an approach for those who have only limited time to devote to this practice, but who also deserve the rewards of this priceless gift. The practice is easily understood and accessible for complete beginners to yoga who have decided that they need a tool to help them balance out everyday pressures. This is the yoga for modern humankind. This practice is for our present-day dilemma: to feel whole and complete while maintaining our day-to-day responsibilities. Kundalini Yoga is a sacred technology that is greatly needed at the present time. It is direct, powerful and simple.

It is important to understand that Kundalini Yoga is concerned with preparing the body for the kundalini energy to rise up through the Sushmana (the energetic spinal column). The scientific aspect of Kundalini Yoga is designed to provide you with the experience of your highest consciousness through the raising of your kundalini. Kundalini is your latent spiritual potential. Through the practice of Kundalini Yoga, this psychic nerve centre is awakened; its revelation is the release of your true potential. For this energy to awaken safely, body and mind need to be strong and able to deal with this very powerful change in consciousness. The practice of Kundalini Yoga is the powerful cleansing of the whole being. Not only do the body and mind need to be cleansed but also the energetic aspects of ourselves. The chakras (energy centres) and meridians (energy pathways) need to be unblocked and activated to allow this new influx of dynamic energy to flow freely throughout the whole being.

Kundalini and chakra work are closely linked. The kundalini energy can be depicted as a serpent, coiled in three and a half turns, sleeping in the Muladhara (Base, or Root, Chakra), the densest of all the chakras. But please note that Yogi Bhajan does not support the concept of kundalini as the coiled serpent, but rather as the blueprint for the full potential of humankind.

Kundalini is known as the spiritual nerve, seated in the base of the spine, waiting to be awakened. With the practice of Kundalini Yoga this nerve can be stimulated and start to become activated as it breaks through the blockage at the Muladhara, travelling upwards through the Sushmana and piercing every chakra along the way, until it reaches the Crown, where full enlightenment is attained.

You do not have to charge in with the intention of raising the kundalini to full enlightenment, although this is the goal of all forms of yoga. There is a more acceptable, more gentle, way of introducing you to the sheer potential that is within you, and showing you how this potential can be released. This method is to gently rouse or stir the kundalini energy in the Ida and Pingala channels, which interweave around the Sushmana, every time you embark on a kundalini kriya. The general pattern of a kundalini kriya is to awaken and build up the Pranic energy. This is then guided to the relevant area that you wish to work on. For example, if your digestive system needs working on, a set to help with decision-making or an emotional state that is upsetting you might be helpful. By directing the energy to a particular chakra, organ, or issue in your life, this blockage will be dissolved and once again you will be back in balance. The negative effects will harm you no more.

There are over 8.4 million kriyas, all designed to deal with the day-to-day challenges we face. There are kriyas for physical issues, such as the digestion, circulation, immune system (disease resistance), lower back problems, glandular malfunctions, menopause and sexuality problems. There are also kriyas for the mind, to clear confusion, addictions, haunting thoughts and creative blocks. Additionally, there are kriyas to balance the emotions, to bring about feelings of ecstasy, to dispel fear and paranoia, to bring about stillness and to attain the empowering ability to accept and forgive all aspects of your life.

Meditation is also a very important part of the practice. This allows the body and mind to process the journey of the kriya. The energy has travelled along a certain pathway, awakening, dispelling and moving your energetic bodies. The meditation process is a lesson in inner awareness. Sometimes the meditation will have a breathing technique to enable the mind to quieten as you turn inwards into the realm of feelings and emotions. When this happens you will be able to observe your thoughts as they come and go. This is the start of the practice known as 'becoming the watcher'. It is through this method that you become master of the mind.

At other times there will be a mantra to accompany the meditation. A mantra is always equipped with a coded sonic vibration that cuts through the psyche and starts to balance out areas within that need attention. When there is a mantra, you may find yourself immersed in the sound. This is the most powerful part of Kundalini Yoga. The word *mantra* breaks down into *man*, which means 'mind' and *tra*, which is 'to vibrate'. Therefore, mantra means 'to vibrate the mind'. This miraculous technique shifts many character traits and behavioural patterns that keep us suffering. In the chapter on Mantra (*see page* 51), I will explain exactly how this sonic science works.

I would like to close this section by saying that you can never predict a kundalini class. It is always full of surprises, since many changes will be going on in all the various people present. There have been times in my classes when there have been outbursts of laughter, which is always good fun and I actively encourage it. Yoga is usually synonymous with seriousness, quiet and solemnity, but this is not always the case. Laughter is common in my classes. It is, after all, an explosion of happiness. This usually happens when a painful emotion or memory has been released. It is also common to find yourself so immersed in the kriya and the breathing that you surface to find tears falling down your cheeks. You may not actually be crying, but tears are falling silently. This is always a very powerful realization of the many changes that are taking place within you.

When you experience this, you will find that harmony and balance are restored to you, and you will feel within an endless supply of energy and happiness. When you experience this, even for a few brief moments, your life will not be the same again. The inner light is now switched on, shining through you, and others will not fail to be drawn towards you. You will become a beacon for humankind, a touchstone for the truth, and the living reality of who we really are.

To everyone who embarks on the path of kundalini, I wish you the greatest journey. May your path show you the many examples of Divinity that are around you at any given moment. May you realize the ultimate truth: that only Love can set you free. Be free, my friend, as it is your birthright.

Be Grateful, BE GREAT *and* BE FULL Yogi Bhajan

The Benefits of Kundalini Yoga

In my experience you can benefit greatly within a minute of starting genuine practice of Kundalini Yoga. There have been many times when I have sat down to begin my practice feeling mentally 'all over the place'. Yet within minutes of starting the kriya, all inner turmoil has dissolved. My mind has even completely settled during the initial tuning-in process.

There have been occasions when I have been angry or full of the most desperate sadness, and yet time and again the miracle of Kundalini Yoga washes away the negativity, so that my own Sun can shine again.

When a feeling or an emotion such as anger or hurt is making itself known to you, then this is the very best time to do your practice. When you become aware of it, half the battle is won. By applying the science of Kundalini Yoga to your everyday experiences, you will begin to master your own destiny.

The acknowledgement of your negative feelings and thoughts is confirmation that you are on the home run. The final part of the process is just a little more work on actually allowing yourself to let go.

Kundalini Yoga will give you the opportunity to achieve a healthy body, a balanced mind and a vast increase in energy manifesting as vitality, creativity and radiance. You may well begin to feel peaceful and strong, ready to meet life's challenges, and win. But if you have not experienced something, how can it be true for you? That is the difference between knowledge and wisdom. Knowledge is something you can acquire after reading a book; wisdom is when you have had the experience for yourself. The real results emerge when you systematically and consciously apply yourself to the practice. Things will begin to fall into place, the Universe will respond to your efforts.

Increased Awareness

Kundalini Yoga is known as 'the yoga of awareness'. One of the first benefits may be an increased sensitivity in your inner awareness. You may begin to uncover and understand many aspects of yourself that were once hidden. It will become increasingly obvious what it is that truly reflects you, and what does not. You will begin to understand what you need to improve in your life, and how you wish your life to be.

Improved Bodily Functions

All your bodily functions will be significantly improved. The cardiovascular, digestive, glandular, respiratory, lymphatic and nervous systems will be given the opportunity to be in good working order.

Flexible Body and Mind

Your flexibility will improve over time; this again will increase energy throughout your body, and help with getting up in the mornings. But it is no good just having a flexible body; the mind needs to be accommodating, in the same way. You will notice a deeper level of patience, understanding of the other people's perspective and a willingness to 'bend' to settle a situation for the good of all.

Stress Reduction

Relaxation techniques have the ability to quieten the mind, giving you a sense of inner peace and stillness. Increased endurance within the nervous system will soothe edgy nerves. You will be able to cope with irritating situations without raising your stress levels. Your threshold to remain calm within the storm will be a gift from a strengthened nervous system.

Expanded Lungs

Due to all the breathing exercises that you carry out in Kundalini Yoga, your lung capacity will expand. Conditions such as asthma and panic attacks may well become a thing of the past. Lung expansion will mean that you will increase your intake of Prana (life force).

A Toned and Strengthened Body

Because of all the physical postures of Kundalini Yoga, your body will quickly become finely tuned. It will become strong and toned. Excess body fat will disappear and structure and shape will begin to take place. You will begin to feel lighter and your self-image will improve.

Cleansing

Yoga and meditation powerfully cleanse us of physical, mental and emotional obstructions, worn-out attitudes and beliefs. This will leave space to develop beneficial and positive new ones that truly reflect us.

Good Health

Because the immune system becomes strengthened, you will have the opportunity to enjoy vibrant good health, and if you become ill you will know how to heal yourself.

Opportunities

You can develop the ability to manifest your deepest desires, and begin to draw opportunities towards you. No longer will life be about fighting for what you want.

Strength of Character

Muscular development is one side-product of strength. What really begin to develop are the qualities of endurance, commitment, the development of the will and faith in your own unlimited potential. You will achieve greater mental clarity and focus. It will become easier to act consistently, to finish tasks and to be truthful and honest.

Beauty

Radiance and the impression that you leave in the hearts of others will be developed. The glandular system is a major player in our sense of well-being. Glandular balance will leave you feeling and looking great. Your demeanour will reflect how you feel inside. You will have the confidence to shine. Your complexion will be youthful and your eyes will sparkle brightly.

Healing

Your healing powers will manifest through your presence, words and touch. One smile from you will uplift a thousand souls.

Well-Being

You may experience an increase in energy, resulting in a ceasing of tiredness or lack of get-up-and-go. Energy will flow through you, unblocked and bringing every aspect of you to life. You will also notice the ability to relax thoroughly, and your sleep will replenish you completely.

Good Decision-Making

Because you will become the master of your life, your decision-making will be in accordance to your true values. Because you will become less emotional, decision-making will be easier. You will be able to initiate change, rather than sit back playing the helpless victim.

Heightened Sensory Awareness

Your intuition will be developed. You will be able to access a set of certainties that you can count on. All your senses will become sharper.

Breaking Addictions and Bad Habits

The need to self-destruct will begin to diminish. You will be given the tools to be able to get to the bottom of the need to over-indulge in drugs, alcohol, sex or food. With an increased awareness of the Self, all your bad habits will begin to fall away.

Attracting the Right Relationship

You will begin to recognize the inner beauty and be attracted to that in a partner rather than repeating the same dysfunctional patterns in a relationship.

Enhancing Sexual Activity

Because you have developed a vital body and soul consciousness the merging of two people will become a deep, joyous, penetrating and radiant sexual pleasure. The act of sex will become an integration of human and Divine energies in pure love.

Increasing Creativity

You will become spontaneous, expressive and your mind will be creative.

Heightening Your Spiritual Sense

You will be able to open your mind to the bigger picture; you will become aware of seeing the goodness in everyone in every situation. *Me* will become *we*. Attitudes such as trust, acceptance, gratitude and non-attachment will become second nature to you.

Opening Your Heart

You will be able to develop the joy of life. Life will become relaxed and fun; you may become 'unreasonably' happy. You will feel taken care of. Even in your darkest moments, there will be joy, as you will know that life is only a drama. With your heart open, you will be in love with life.

A Drugless High

Along with exercises to break addictions and to repair the damages of drug abuse, this book offers exercises that will quickly and easily alter your consciousness. You will receive extraordinary effects from many of the sets and meditations. In Kundalini Yoga you can experience all the same effects as taking drugs, but without suffering any loss of character and values or mental and physiological damage. In my opinion, drugs and other mind-altering substances give you the illusion of an expansion in consciousness, whereas Kundalini Yoga delivers the real thing.

Yogi Bhajan

Harbhajan Singh Puri was born on 26 August 1929 in Kot Harkaran, formerly India, now Pakistan. Yogi Bhajan mastered Kundalini Yoga by the time he was 16. During his youth he studied with many masters, including the Mahan Tantric of that time, Sant Hazara Singh, who was also a master of Kundalini Yoga.

At the present time Yogi Bhajan is the only recognized living Master of Kundalini Yoga. He is also the Chief Minister of Sikh Dharma in the West and the Mahan Tantric of White Tantric Yoga. This is a very powerful form of tantric yoga practised in pairs, to deeply cleanse the sub-conscious mind.

In 1969 Yogi Bhajan came to America, his mission statement being 'I have come to create teachers, not gather disciples'. With this humble intention, this is exactly what he is doing.

Yogi Bhajan is my type of spiritual master, happily walking through life with a sense of Self ever-present. He has a finely tuned sense of humour and packs a mean punch when it comes to letting us all know about ourselves and the crazy games that we play. I have included here a lecture (*see page* 19) that he gave in 2000 so that you can really feel the essence of this inspiring man.

I love the driving force of his teachings; his encouragement keeps me going even when I feel beaten. He inspires, elevates and gives strength to all who cross his path. It is these gifts that I have adapted to my own approach. Yogi Bhajan has shown me that we can all go far beyond what we think we are capable of. When we prove this to ourselves the sense of exhilaration and self-achievement can change our life and our perception of our Self forever.

The other wonderful thing about Yogi Bhajan is his ability to be a spiritual master to the masses.

Due to his rising popularity, he was invited to teach at the spectacular Atlanta Music Festival in 1970. At that time there were many casualties from the 1960s attending class, after deciding to quit their various addictions and the accompanying hedonistic lifestyle.

He was a great success in Los Angeles in the 1970s and many 'hotshot' students came to class. But he knew that his path did not lie with celebrities. His mission was to create teachers. So the first thing he did was to ask all the students to take a raw garlic supplement. The celebrities vanished almost overnight.

Yogi Bhajan still has many contacts within celebrity circles, but he chooses not to cater to them. He has met many of the people who hold temporal and spiritual power on the planet, but his mission is to bring Kundalini Yoga in its perfection to the people who hear the inner calling.

The Self-Sensory System of The Aquarian Age

BY YOGI BHAJAN, PH.D, FROM A LECTURE GIVEN 1 AUGUST 2000

In the next 12 to 14 years you will be needed by the world. It does not matter who one is today, or to whom one belongs; peoples' minds are going to go empty.

In the Piscean Age, the main need was for knowledge, for creative legacy. That's why in the Piscean Age sex was taboo; it was monitored, matured, glorified. Sex and Sensuality were considered the primary attractions. Beauty was physical, and people pursued each other. Sexual intercourse was the orientation of relationship, and it reached the point of obnoxious duality; perversion became very prominent.

But the time is changing; people are looking towards fulfilment of the Self through purity and piety, individuality, and reality. They don't want to practise duality any more. Sex will not be the attraction. A sensory system in which the individual will find him or herself complete.

Communication will be humongous. Everybody will have access to all knowledge. With the push of a button you will get all knowledge that you want. The obsession with sex will have no place. One will not look for satisfaction through physical inter-course anymore. One will find satisfaction through the self-sensory system, which will be delivered in the next 50 years. The foundations are being laid because the cusp period is 1991 to 2012 for the Age of Pisces to go and for the Age of Aquarius to come. We have already gone through nine of these 21 years.

What is the personal sensory system? There will be no need for cosmetic makeup. People will be open, straight, simple and their beauty will be internal, not external. Men and women are going to reach out with such dignity, such devotion, such an elevated, loftiness of self, and the beauty of the human character will be so bewitching, not only will the ones who are willing be enjoying and realizing, but also their realization will be so profound that no destructive temptation by another person will work.

The Piscean Age was the ugliest age – an era in which the female was rooted out from her roots and exploited to the brink and to the brim by men. The male/female relationship didn't have any strength. It didn't have any character. It didn't have any taste. So females in the past century gave birth to some of the most fearful, insecure, impotent, or oversexed men, and sexual disorder was worse than ever before in the past 3,000 years.

The men whom you called great in the last century wanted to indulge in the power of destruction. That's why we created the atom bomb, the hydrogen bomb, smart bombs, we had two wars, and we killed more people in the name of religion than anything else. And religion did not become reality, but an ugly fanaticism.

The ironic thing that happened in the last century is that man started finding God outside himself. Man forgot that God is the working God, 'Karta Purkh', which

Nanak, the first Sikh Guru, said works and breathes in us. It's part of us, it's not separate. We were blind to God's presence everywhere.

Today we have become limited, small, squeezed to a point of just physical existence. We have little quality, quantity, character and commitment. Our character is mostly inconsistent. We often say things that are not true. We truthfully say things that are not true. We dramatically say things that are not true.

We do the most detrimental things on this planet. In order to build a tower that surrounds the individual – like adding to how many houses, how many boyfriends, how much money we have – we end up on dirt, a termite heap of dirt.

When a race of humans starts making a mockery of themselves openly and obnoxiously, nothing is sacred. So this is the state of affairs, and it has to go on for 12 more years of this cusp period.

And it will be bad for us.

My idea to present this to you is that many of you will try to reach out to help people or to help yourselves, and you will have something to understand. It's called 'building the foundation of the New Age'.

The Age of Aquarius will be the age of experience in which the people of experience will be liked, respected, worshipped, talked to and understood. It's not a matter of how old you are or how young you are or how white you are or how black you are.

Religion, as it has been known, has become absolutely obsolete. In the past 5000 years religion has been teaching you how to redeem your soul. The soul is already redeemed. What you should redeem is your being not true to your words, not true to your commitment, not true to your character. That's what you should redeem.

The fact is there is nothing more beautiful, more worthy, or more conscious than you.

The time has come for self-value. And the question is not 'To be or not to be' but 'I AM, I am'. The time has come not to search for God, but to be God. The time is not to worship God, but to trust and dwell in the working God.

As this is coming through me, it is cleansing me. If you are not listening and only hearing, you are not getting it. But if you are listening, it will go into you. You have to come to the awareness of how bad and unfortunate it is that we have made this world as ugly as possible – and how beautiful, actually, God created it. We are purely enemies of God, because God within us is in pain, and there is no God outside us. Each one is the manifestation of God, so it won't work to create God by making a stone God. Every grain of sand is God.

Those who hustle and hassle and move and want will suffer. They will not get what they want. Now the time has come that we will have a meditative mind to wait and see what comes to us. Our minds will direct us to work towards the right channels. And we will meet the right people.

Our future is now, and our presence is our purity. We don't have to purify ourselves; we are pure. We simply have to stop making it ugly by diversion, by concoctions, by stories, and by creating meaningless romance and fantasy, and imagining things that are zero. We'll master ourselves through our service, through our character, through our commitment, and through the powerful thing that we have – our grace. Our individual grace is our most wanted quality today. And our projection, which will give us satisfaction, fulfilment, and exaltation, is our nobility. We will act nobly, graciously, kindly, and compassionately. These are our essential features.

Our creativity will be our sensory system. And through this sensory system we will be overflowing with energy, touching the hearts of people and feeling their feeling, and filling their emptiness. We will act gratefully and our flow will fulfil the grateful-ness in the hearts of others. It will be a new relationship. We will create a new humanity that will have the new sensory system, and through this we will establish the Age of Aquarius. This is the fundamental character you have to learn by heart.

The Age of Aquarius

We are living in very interesting times, and they are going to become even more interesting. This time will become a marked point in the history of the Universe and of Humankind. We are witnessing the dawn of a new age, moving from the Age of Pisces into the Age of Aquarius. Many religious and spiritual teachers have prophesied this time, and now astrological and scientific leaders are confirming its existence.

It is generally agreed that the actual time that we enter the Age of Aquarius will be 2012. This is backed up by many spiritual teachers and those in the scientific field. In 1961 science discovered, through the use of satellites, what is now known as the 'photon belt'. This is a belt of photon energy particles, the result of a collision between anti-electrons and electrons. This split-second collision causes both electron energies to cancel on impact, and the result of the impact is to form photon energy.

This photon belt is a result of mass annihilation between both types of electrons, and it promises to be a major source of energy in the very near future.

This time of transition from one age to another will bring turbulent times; it will lead to an increased rate of change in our society and ourselves. This shift involves nothing less than a major review of our world views and our consciousness.

We need to learn a way to be happy and to thrive under this new pressure. This entry into a new belt of energy will change our rate of vibration to a much higher frequency, to synchronize with that of the Heart Chakra.

This increased rate of change will force people to adapt to this new pace of life, and then master this new era in a short time. Our own eyes have already witnessed this pressure all around us, in our families, and in friends and ourselves. There is personal breakdown and information overload. The limitation of the brain to handle this new information and the awakened sensitivity in our consciousness will exert considerable pressure on us all.

As we cross the threshold of the New Age, leaving behind the dregs of the Piscean Age, we have a choice: make the giant leap of faith to synchronize with the new vibration and realize our best hopes and dreams, or to cling to the past, to stay with what we know. In the Aquarian Age we will enjoy union with all humankind, elitism will break down and a sense of connection between all men and women will be experienced. There will also be a need for responsibility, both individually and collectively, to create the environment that truly reflects our ideals. No more will we be looking outside for God or self-worth, but instead we will realize that we are God, and our sense of self-worth is in abundance within us all.

The science of Kundalini Yoga is available at just the right time to help us master the mental discipline necessary to change old habits in the subconscious mind and amplify perception of, and sensitivity to, the subtle energies produced by thought. By acknowledging this process and accepting its validity, we can exercise a positive influence over our lives and collectively, on the environment, through our mental bodies.

Collective human disgraces such as hunger, homelessness, rape, war, racism and pollution of the environment will end. For the suffering of one is the suffering of all.

A Comparison Between the Piscean and Aquarian Ages

QUOTES BY YOGI BHAJAN FROM A LECTURE HE GAVE IN LOS ANGELES ON 14 AUGUST 1987
ON THE HARMONIC CONVERGENCE

As we move through these two ages, we will begin to dissolve the perception of duality. No more will there be good and bad, light and dark, right and wrong: instead there will just be.

This may resonate with you, this continuous shifting from one state of mind to the other, and really that's how it's going to be as we play out the effects of duality (pairs of opposites), which was the very nature of Pisces. Aquarius is about throwing off duality and being one with all that is. And with that in mind, every time you feel you have slipped off the path and are in darkness let me remind you, 'you never slip off the path, the path is both light and dark, it's the continuous journey'. But the greater reality is that if we continue to label the darkness as bad times, we are still thinking in a mode of duality. There are no bad times, there is no darkness, your life, just is.

Pisces	Aquarius
Ideals	
Faith, hope	Knowing, choosing, doing
Everyone loves a winner	We are all winners
Personal achievement	Self-respect
Competition	Co-operation
Relationships	
Romance, passion, conditional love	Heart-centred, responsive to change unconditional love
Parasitic, partnerships, binding	Independence, individualism, freedom
Life	
Romance, glamour, escapism, pursuit of pleasure	Creating heaven on earth, sharing, creative, following the heart
Heroes, stars, rulers, followers	Freedom from elitism

The Myths and Mysteries

There are so many mysteries surrounding kundalini, it can very difficult to grasp what it is and, more importantly, to discover the truth regarding raising the kundalini. *Kundal* translates as 'coil of', and *ini* translates as 'endearment'. The full translation is 'the coil in the hair of the beloved'.

When you are reading about kundalini, be sure to keep an open mind, as many writers on the subject are describing something they may not necessarily have experienced. Although their intentions are well meant, it is worth noting that many misrepresentations do not lead back to a kundalini yoga master, but to a rumour or a misconception.

A warning about a technique is valueless as it only creates insecurity and misunderstanding. A negative opinion may prevent the freedom to explore; only your own experience will be your truth.

Watch out for masters who openly demonstrate their psychic powers before an audience. A real master will repeatedly encourage students to turn their attention away from the teacher and in towards themselves.

You need to know your teacher's credentials; the power of kundalini is the force within the atom. This is not a subject to be taken lightly; it requires reverence and the utmost respect. If it is your intention to activate your kundalini, I wholeheartedly recommend that you take up the practice of Kundalini Yoga as taught by Yogi Bhajan. Please be aware of this and ask your teacher if you are not sure.

Under this form of practice you will be under the umbrella of his energetic guidance, secure in the knowledge that it is a tried-and-tested method. A kundalini experience is simply the experience of awakening.

Here is a passage in Yogi Bhajan's words about how you raise the kundalini:

> *It is easy to awaken the Kundalini, but it is very difficult to take it to the Crown. It requires a great deal of perseverance, purity and steady practice. Students feel they have reached the goal just because they get some mystic experience or psychic powers. This is a sad mistake. Full realization alone can give the final liberation, perfect peace and highest bliss.*
>
> *You must generate the pressure of the Prana (incoming life force) and mix it with the Apana (eliminating force), and thus, when the two join together, you generate heat ('tapa') in the Navel Centre. With this heat of the Prana, you put a pressure or charge on the Kundalini, the soul nerve, which is coiled in three and half circles. This will awaken it so that it may pierce through the chakras until the energy comes to the Crown at the top of the head.*
>
> *Once you have raised it, that's it. The hardest job is to keep it up, to keep the channels clean and clear.*
>
> YOGI BHAJAN

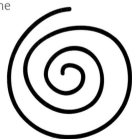

So, really the idea is to bring the energy up from the base of the spine up through the whole energetic system to the crown. As the energy raises it pierces through every chakra, activating their positive attributes within the individual. When the energy comes into the head it will activate the pineal gland to start secreting, and so bring about a major change in consciousness. The phenomena attached to the raising of Kundalini should not be the goal; otherwise you will just become sidetracked.

My interpretation of kundalini is that it is an energy, which when activated reveals to you your true potential. Have you ever had a moment when you felt untouchable, huge and powerful, like an eagle? Well, that is kundalini. It is the full creative potential of humankind. Kundalini is always flowing through us. If it wasn't we could not remain alive. But there is a vast reservoir in the fourth vertebrae, which when tapped into can change our consciousness. There is a very simple diagram that depicts the simplicity of it all. When you compare it to the ancient symbol, the Caduceus, you can see clear similarities. You may well have come across this symbol before as it is the well-known symbol of the medical profession. In the chapter on the chakras (*see page* 82) I will explain in detail what this diagram refers to. But in the meantime, the staff represents our central nerve that is within the spinal column, while the two serpents are the two nerve channels that twine around the spinal cord. In esoteric teachings the left nerve is named Ida, while the right is named Pingala, and the spinal column is known as the Sushmana. The reason the symbol depicts serpents is because in mythology the serpent represents knowledge. Kundalini is nearly always understood as serpentine, but that is just a metaphor.

The idea is to bring the energy up from the base of the spine, through the whole energetic system, to the Crown. As the energy rises, it pierces through every chakra, activating the positive attributes of each within the individual. When the energy comes into the head it activates the pineal gland to start secreting, and so bring about a major change in consciousness. It is important to add that the phenomena attached to the raising of kundalini should not be your goal; otherwise you will just become side-tracked.

Once the kundalini energy has been raised, keeping it in the higher centres is a mission in itself. Every word, thought and deed has the ability instantly to lower or raise kundalini. It is as if we are registering our every moment on the most delicate and sensitive thermometer. We need to monitor ourselves constantly, otherwise the kundalini will drop into the lower chakras. If that happens, do not worry, but bear in mind that raising it up will require intentional work on yourself, perhaps necessitating a look at why it dropped in the first place. But, above all else, remember that life is fun and just enjoy the journey.

Is Kundalini Dangerous?

Many Kundalini Yoga warnings come from the Chinese systems, the practitioners of which think that kundalini is a Prana. However, it is kundalini that *organises* the Pranic flows and uses the essence, or Soul, of the being. It can never cause a problem. It is You. The You within You.

Awakened, it expresses you at all levels of subtlety from earth to ether. It is just an energy, which can be used for total consciousness. There are people who state that raising kundalini is troublesome and dangerous, but this is usually because they have not done the hard work required, through the practise of Kundalini Yoga. It is crucial that this is done. The lower chakras have to be cleared of troublesome issues through the full system of yoga. People who tell you of nightmarish experiences have usually had the kundalini experience through either a spontaneous awakening, drug taking, intense meditation, sitting in the presence of a spiritual master or through some other form of spiritual practice. I do not wish to condemn other ways of doing it, but it is my experience that practising Kundalini Yoga, as taught by Yogi Bhajan, will allow you to achieve this goal safely and sensibly.

How Long will it Take?

It will happen when you are ready. Yogi Bhajan has stated that with pure and steadfast practice it is possible to achieve it within 40 days.

Do you need to be Celibate?

No. In Kundalini Yoga it is understood that we have responsibilities and that we are present in the modern world. To be celibate usually means to be by yourself and denying the most powerful urge known to humankind. Yogi Bhajan recommends that once a month is adequate for sexual intercourse with your partner. This may seem a tall order, but it needs to be understood that he is recommending that we conserve the exchange of sexual fluids. You can become intimate with your partner as often as you like, but try to refrain from orgasm or ejaculation. If you do choose to be celibate, remember to practise Sat Kriya every day to utilize the abundance of energy.

Will I get Visions or Psychic Experiences?

This is just the glitter at the bottom of the ladder. This is not the kundalini. It is just the adjustment of your Pranic bodies and nervous system.

Why is the Technology being Shared Now?

The practice of Kundalini Yoga has only been taught publicly since 1969; until then it remained secret. The yogis guarded the knowledge, selectively passing it on by word of mouth. They were selective only because knowledge gives you power, and power can corrupt. It is now time to openly practise this powerful and direct path to transformation. These techniques belong to the people who practise them; it is the heritage of humankind. Future generations will need this technology to stay mentally healthy and physically strong, as we evolve into a new age.

A Kundalini Experience

This is my account, taken from my journal, of the kundalini awakening I was blessed to receive on Monday, 13 July 1999.

The set was on the pineal gland. After each posture, I began to notice an increasingly obvious tingling in my spine, which was very pleasant and for me this confirmed that I was working hard and clearly moving my energy. After a particularly challenging posture, which involved raising my arms above my head for a certain period of time, I noticed a warm 'liquid' rush down my arms into my neck and shoulders. As this happened heat began to 'melt away' my spine. I can only describe that it felt as if the structure of my spine disappeared, I felt as if I had no backbone. This was great. I wasn't bothered at all by this feeling; it did not distract me at all and I just carried on with the next exercise. I was totally enjoying the experience, but wasn't engrossed with the symptoms. I continued to focus on what I was doing. Aware of everything, yet focused on something.

During the meditation, I was aware that I was in what I understood to be the nucleus of the Universe. I then became aware of a shore or an edge of this nucleus; I felt I was at God's feet or shore. There was a distinct awareness of this other form and me: two separate entities. I felt so close to this source, this immense power. It was like standing next to an amplifier at a rock concert. No sound was coming out, just the throb or hum of power. I heard this physically in my ears, I even felt the vibration all over my body, particularly in my heart. It was incredibly powerful.

I remember bowing down to this presence, this throb and pulse of unknowable existence. I realized I was at the Source of all life, I was witnessing God, but still feeling separate.

As I bowed down I forgave myself for every misdeed I had ever done, I forgave myself for hurting others, I forgave those who had hurt me, I forgave everyone for everything. My whole life flashed up before me, other lives passed by, ones I didn't recognize, and faces I had never seen.

All emotions rose to the surface and I observed them slide by as I let them go. Sadness, jealousy, rejection, manipulation, greed, selfishness, anger, aloneness and then finally immense and overwhelming joy, peace and love, so much love. I rose up with tears in my eyes, I looked at God with a complete open heart and with so much gratitude I bowed again and gave my heart to God. I took my heart from myself and surrendered it to God. I was no longer on the shore, and I was now in the nucleus. I had merged with this being. I was at one. My identity did not exist any more. I was still aware, but at that moment I was at one with everything.

When I eventually finished the meditation, I opened my eyes to find tears flowing down my face. My top was drenched in tears, I was glowing, I was radiating, and I felt divinely happy and very excited. I left the class and did not say a word to anyone about it, because, simply, I could not find the words to explain. I could not stop smiling, I just wanted to love everyone, I wanted to scream from the top of the hills, I am not sure what I wanted to say. I was ecstatic.

During the whole of this experience, I want to confirm that there was no fear, no trauma, no nightmarish situations, just the urge to surrender. I believe the choice was there for me, was I going to throw off my ego and become one, or was I going to stay on the shore remaining separate? I believe if I had remained at the edge, the kundalini would not have gone to the very top. Humility was the key that allowed me to experience the absolute awareness of myself. This is simply, God.

The Conclusion

Through the practice of Kundalini Yoga I was able to safely and gently experience the kundalini awakening. I am aware that I was under the energetic guidance of Yogi Bhajan, with a tried-and-tested technique.

I remember prior to the experience that it was a very intense time as I moved through my lower chakras and released various blockages and stale energy. I started yoga for the first time in September 1998, so until July 1999 it was a journey of pure discovery of myself. It still is, but that particular time was a roller coaster of major ups and downs. But I knew what I was doing, I knew who I wanted to be and I was very happy for my life to be examined at last. I was experiencing very intense dreams, mood swings, unexplainable phenomena were happening daily, *but* nothing worried me. It was just my journey through the process. When the experience eventually came, I was ready to experience the most pleasurable and ecstatic event in my life.

There is nothing dangerous about raising the kundalini under the practice of Kundalini Yoga as taught by Yogi Bhajan. The only danger is to get side-tracked by symptoms of what the practice may reveal to you. This is not the goal; only liberation can set you free. It is a journey that we all have to take eventually, to completely free ourselves of the illusion of our everyday lives.

What Does it Feel Like?

It is an overwhelming feeling of pure love and pure joy. It is an upward and outward wave of gratitude, love and peace for all living things. Time momentarily stops; there is nothing other than Union with all of existence. Words alone cannot come close to explaining how it really is. When you too experience it, you will know this.

Raising your kundalini is the experience of awakening to your soul, which knows no limits or boundaries. The soul is the essence of pure love. How can that be dangerous? It is the mind that is our jailer, yet within us all is the key to freedom. But first the hard work needs to be done, and you have to address the clearing of your chakras. Unfortunately no one can escape this.

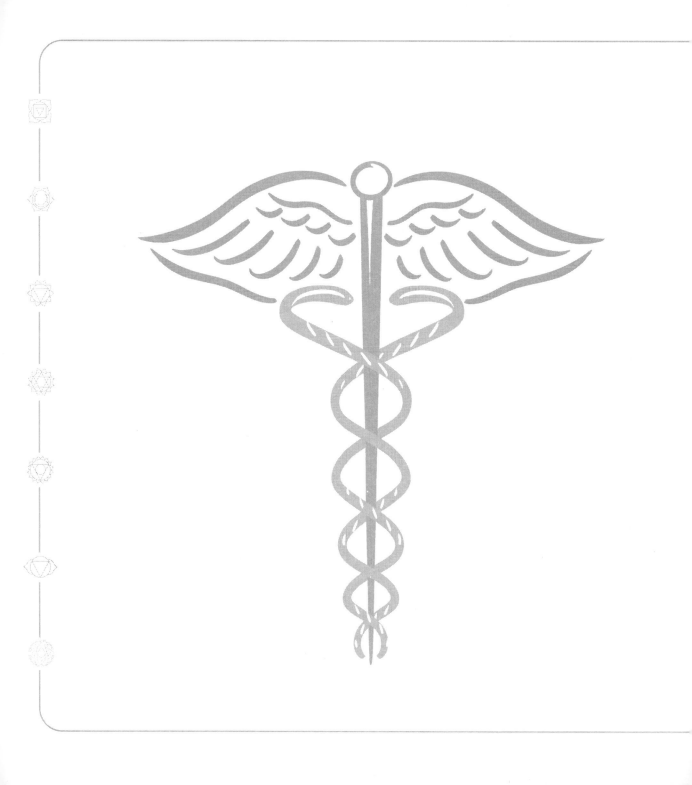

part two

The Science of
Kundalini Yoga

The Three Levels of Being

First we have to acknowledge that we have a three-fold structure. We have three parts to ourselves, not just one, and we need to acquire an in-depth understanding of every part. The first part is the physical *body*, which we tend to understand as our 'real self'. It is not and this is one of our biggest illusions. Scientists inform us that if we compressed our body into a solid lump, it would be no bigger than a thumbnail. We tend to think of ourselves as being this huge, solid body, yet 70% of this body is water; the same ratio as for the planet.

The body serves as a vehicle for us to travel around in through life. It is a very complicated and subtle piece of transport. It has glands, blood circulation, heart-beat pulsation, a brain, sensory apparatus and a complex nervous system. All these systems interweave within a structure of flesh and bone, which make up what we see as being a person.

This physical system is so sensitive that if it is not looked after properly it will start to affect our capacity for life. When we are young we can play mischief with the body, but in old age the body makes us pay for this. The body will record the results of all our actions. Just like a car, the body needs routine maintenance, and unfortunately we cannot change models after a couple of years. We have only one body and we need to take the utmost care of it.

The *mind* is the next important part of our three-fold structure. We often become a slave to the mind, as it becomes the master, and we blindly follow. We need to change the balance of who masters who. In the first place the mind is there to allow us to think and analyse, and then make choices about our conclusions. But we have lost the knowledge of our mind and how to work together with this part of ourselves. The mind often behaves like a mischievous child, seeing how far it can push us. We often get confused into thinking that we are the mind. We think that all our thoughts must be true, because after all, we are thinking them.

The mind guides our actions and reactions. Everything depends on our mental outlook. The problem is, as we think, so we are. If somebody is beautiful or ugly to us, it is a result of our mental evaluation. All of our experience in life is filtered through the mind. Happy and unhappy belong to our mind, not to the world. We must learn to understand how powerful the mind is; we attract all that comes to us just by the power of thought. Keep your thoughts positive, uplifting and full of love and forgiveness and then just sit back and watch how your life will begin to reflect what you are thinking. Stay mindful and begin to watch your thoughts, without reacting to them. This is one of the most powerful ways to take mastery of the mind.

The third, important, part of our three-fold structure is the *Soul*, the spirit. As no lamp can burn without fuel, so no life can exist without a relationship to the spirit within. The soul contains our message and our mission; it holds the key to who we are, and how to become who we are. But where is this soul? The soul sits within our heart. This is not the organ itself, but the very inner core of ourselves.

Happiness and mastery of the spiritual is a simple and direct practice. The problem is that we have never opened our minds to know our origin; it just draws a blank every time we ask the question 'where do I come from?'.

The answer is group consciousness. The power of the group has more leverage than an individual. The group will continuously reflect your Self back to you. When you have spiritual longing, it is because you are experiencing your Self as separate, and you feel, or rather know, that there is more, there is something that will take this loneliness away. Take care of your spiritual factor by joining with others to experience and elevate your Self. When we practise by ourselves, there will always be lack of knowledge, lack of a teacher. Ego, fear and karma will become barriers, which will keep a person limited. The development of group consciousness into the experience of Infinity is the bridge to universal consciousness. It releases the unlimited Self and fulfils the spiritual longing.

Your basic human structure is your three-fold nature and the relationship of you, the finite, and the temporary with the wholeness, the Infinite, the permanent. God is not separate from you; the source from which you came is within you. This is the fundamental framework through which we function and experience our life. As you practise Kundalini Yoga you will grow. Like a snake, you will shed old skins to become more of who you are. You will need to examine certain attitudes, behaviours and emotional habits. But it will be empowering. You will begin to see and understand all the patterns in your life, the reasons why you did what you did. You will no longer run around in circles getting out of breath and getting nowhere. Instead there will be answers, and from your understanding you will acquire the ability to change. There are several challenges to confront. Your mind must be developed, artistic and self-controlled. It needs to be neutral, allowing you to enjoy the constant change that is within life. You learn as a child that you are an individual and that you want to control everything. You want sunshine all the time. No one can live with sunshine all the time; the real beauty of life is based on constant shades between light and dark. We need both the light and the dark, the push and the pull of life, to know exactly where we stand. Good health is another challenge. We all want good health. Without this it is difficult to work on other aspects of our lives. There are two types of sickness: intentional and unintentional. Intentional sickness is when you know that what you are doing will lead to sickness, but you continue to threaten your health anyway. Unintentional sickness is when you are ignorant about the effects of what you are doing or when you are subject to powerful external forces.

Kundalini Yoga teaches you the techniques and awareness to stay healthy. You will gain a strong immune system, vital glands, a strong nervous system, good circulation and an awareness of the impact of your habits. This foundation within the body will let you deal with the mental and spiritual facets of your life.

To make use of yoga in its totality, you have to know what living is. You have to know what a relationship is and what values this life can give you. If you know what you want, then you can find it. But first, you must decide what it is you are doing this for, what you are aspiring to, what you want to become. Through meditation you can calm the mind, but when you close your eyes where are you going to go?

Kundalini Yoga develops your relationship with your mental potential. You learn to use the clarity of the Neutral Mind. You begin to sharpen your intellect and avoid using it to create self-doubt or insecurity. Every student of Kundalini Yoga has to confront insecurity and self-doubt. Powerful feelings of insecurity can create problems and disrupt happiness. Kundalini Yoga, meditation and white tantra will all work on disentangling the threads of insecurity from the layers of the subconscious. In every mental state the subconscious plays a major role that we are unaware of. We all think we know our 'past', though actually there is no past. Our 'past' is our experience in our subconscious mind. We become so attached to that, and it is that attachment that prevents us moving forwards. We always look back to the past for answers and guidance – let it go, it does not exist.

In Kundalini Yoga we 'cook' this sub-conscious mind, make a tasty meal out of it and then eat it.

There is one more pattern that we all confront in Kundalini Yoga. We often hold a feeling that we are very limited and small. This is our self-belittlement. We play this game very well, and there are three ways to play it. We can either play it to get sympathy from another person, or we play it to become recognized, or sometimes we play it so well that we actually feel it and are fooled. We all do it. It is just a question of degree. Kundalini Yoga dissolves our self-belittlement and replaces it with self-celebration.

In Kundalini Yoga the most important thing is *experience*. The experience will go right into the depths of your heart. *Understanding* is only the wrapping paper that contains the full potential of the gift I am passing on to you.

The Ten Bodies

The ten bodies are our ten layers of consciousness. These ten layers make up our subtle anatomy; our energetic blueprint, the map of how our energy flows. A healthy, vibrant person has an energy field extending two and three-quarter metres (nine feet) beyond the physical body. This is what we are aiming to achieve. When our energetic field falls below one metre (three feet), this is when we encounter trouble in our lives. Within the ten bodies we have one Physical Body, three mental bodies (Negative, Positive and Neutral) and six subtle bodies. All of these layers are vibrating at higher frequencies, therefore becoming finer and more subtle.

As you practise yoga so you clean out these bodies, and strengthen the flow of energy within them. This, in turn, will make you 'shine' with radiance, your energy will extend and people will not be able to help being attracted to you.

Out of the ten, two bodies will always remain; the Soul and the Subtle Body. These contain your true essence, the core of who you are. The others dissolve at the moment of death. The Soul and the Subtle Body continue.

The energy of the subtle anatomy is Prana; this is the substance that makes the atom move. It is the basis of Creation. It is also known as 'life force', astral light or chi.

The Soul Body

The first body is the Soul Body. What is the Soul? It is the point of light, the Infinite aspect of us. It is the part of us that never dies, and it holds our mission and message. When we connect with our Soul we consciously awaken to our journey. It is when we become aware that we are the 'Atma' (Soul) and we are all part of the 'Paramatma' (Universal Soul). In several scriptures it is known that we have 84 million lifetimes, and it is the Atma that keeps coming back to learn more about what it means to be human.

The Negative Mind

The function of the Negative Mind is to signal inherent danger and to protect you from possible harm. If the Negative Mind is disordered, you will see only the negative aspect of every situation. This could lead to you becoming isolated from others, as you will be paralysed by fear at the prospect of life and be unable to take control. The Negative Mind has blind spots. An example of this is when people keep repeating the same pattern over and over again without learning the lesson of their mistakes. Their Negative Mind has a blind spot to that particular behavioural trait, and therefore understanding becomes impossible. 'Fight or flight' is an aspect of the Negative Mind.

The Positive Mind

The Positive Mind shows you the lesson and the best possible outcome of the situation. This aspect of the mind needs to be encouraged and listened to. This is the part of the mind that encourages optimism, excitement, enthusiasm, it is the 'get up and go' feeling and the rise to the challenge. If the Positive Mind is overlooked, its energy may become eroded and the Negative Mind will begin to take over. However, there is a danger of living too fully in the positive mind, as an imbalance would lead to over-optimism, an absence of clear thinking or of being an 'idiot' in a situation.

The Neutral Mind

The Neutral Mind weighs the information from the other two, and then it makes a decision. The Neutral Mind does not have regrets or guilt. The Neutral Mind just is. It is conscious decision-making. To forgive you need to be in the Neutral Mind. It is the mind that is known as the 'yogic mind'. It is the stillness, the peace and the grace. It is this state of mind that the practice of yoga amplifies

The Physical Body

The Physical Body allows us to participate fully in life. The lesson of the Physical Body is balance. The quality of the Physical Body is sacrifice and communication. A person with a weak Fifth Body is someone who is shy and afraid to come out of themselves, while a person with a powerful Fifth Body is enthusiastic about everything that they do. Self-sacrifice and the ability to endure pain are hallmarks of a strong Fifth Body.

The Arc Line

The Arc Line is the circuit of energy that runs from ear to ear. You can clearly see this depicted in religious paintings as the 'halo'. The Arc Line represents your sense of intuition, justice and, like the Negative Mind, will warn you of possible dangers, but from an energetic source. It will protect you from negative energy. Women have two Arc Lines; the other one is located between the nipples.

If you have a powerful Arc Line, you will be able to receive energy from the Cosmos. You will not have to read books to acquire information, as you will be able to access it through meditation. The Arc Line communicates who you are to other people, without a word being spoken.

The Auric Body

This encases the whole of the Physical Body. The aura is made up of electromagnetic energy. The electric aspect is the male energy, while the magnetic is the female energy. It is a protective shell that makes you sensitive to external and internal stimuli. It continuously changes, as you feel yourself moving from one emotion to the other. It is like a sea of light and colour. A person who can see auras will be able to see your state of health and mind. As we interact with other people, so our auras will either blend or deflect. A person who is loving and peaceful will naturally attract us, and we, too, will start to feel the same way. An angry person will cause us to be repelled, and we will turn away. Unless of course you are an angry person, where, instead, it will attract you because you will recognize the same aura. You see this happening when fights and violence break out between people.

The Pranic Body

This is the energy of the whole body in motion. This energy keeps the heart beating, the blood and diaphragm moving and controls the metabolic rate and temperature. For this body to really give you what it is capable of you have to breathe properly (long, deep breathing), into the diaphragm. It is there that you connect with yourself, and release the storehouse of Pranic energy. The Pranic Body gives you energy, courage, control over your mind and healing power.

The Subtle Body

This is known as the 'cosmic egg'. All the events of all your life are stored here. There are two bodies that stay with you constantly: the Soul and the Subtle Body. The Soul and the Subtle Body come in to the being at the same time, and they leave together at the moment of death.

The Subtle Body allows you to discern the subtlety of life, helping you to understand the dynamics of a situation. You will be able to learn new things easily, such as new skills. You will be able to tune in to a situation and understand the things that are not being said. You will also be able to interpret and analyse easily, using just a small amount of energy.

The Radiant Body

The Radiant Body gives you radiance and a powerful presence. The strength of the Radiant Body will give you courage in the face of any obstacle. Positive things will be drawn to you. People with a powerful Radiant Body seem to shine with an inner glow. There is a strength that attracts people and a feeling of trust and integrity that enables them to love and be loved.

The Mind

We have one thousand thoughts per second; some that we acknowledge and the majority that we do not. Only a few thoughts go on to produce emotions, and these emotions can go in two directions. Either they become devotion or commotion. Devotion is where there is no sadness and no pain. The mind is bewitched with happiness and contentment; we are happy in our world. Commotion can, by contrast, lead to patterns, and these patterns govern the mind. We call these patterns habits. The task of the yogi is to balance the mental functions to gain a clear perspective of what is real and what is not. Because we are wrapped in layers of mental and emotional habits that cloud our perception, we then go on to make choices that are against our own Self. When we do that we are asleep. We view the moment of choice through the blinkers of the ego. As the mind becomes refined, judgement also improves and we go on to make consistent decisions that bring happiness and growth.

It is very important to have a positive mental attitude. We are what we think and feel. The way we think and feel sets up currents in the astral plane, which then go on to create what it is that we have thought. We can use positive thoughts to bring us what we want. Our negative thoughts can go on to create our own worst nightmares. All we have to do to take charge of our lives is to discipline the mind.

Mastering the mind is one of the aims of Kundalini Yoga. Liberation is the experience of your own Infinity, and that lies far beyond the realms of the mind. What we need to do is sharpen the mind, make it clearer and make it serve us. The key to taking control of the mind is the breath. The mind will always follow the breath, and the body will always follow the mind. When you are in complete gridlock with the mind, look at the body. It will no doubt be rigid and full of tension. Just start long, deep breathing, and observe how the mind begins to slow down and how the body starts to relax.

If we do not know how to slow the mind, if we are constantly going over things in the head, the body will be so tense that we will be blocking the circulation of our energy. There will be dis-harmony within us. Being in gridlock with the mind can cause serious problems.

Slowing the mind is one thing, but the real goal of all yoga is to strengthen and develop the Neutral Mind.

We have three levels in the mind: The Conscious Mind (Negative, Positive and Neutral Minds), the subconscious and the unconscious mind being the deepest level of the mental realm.

The Conscious Mind

The Conscious Mind has already been covered in the chapter on the ten bodies (*see page* 41). This is the everyday mind, the part that analyses and makes choices based on received conscious stimuli. It is our decision-making; judgement and understanding of all the various situations that cross our path.

The Subconscious Mind

This is the second level of the mind. It is very simply the mental 'in' tray. The Conscious Mind is just the tip of the iceberg; most of what motivates us is way below the surface. A great proportion of our behaviour is dictated to us by our subconscious, but it does not have the ability to separate fact from fiction. It is a vast container of all our thoughts, words and feelings that we receive constantly. It cannot process what it receives: it just collects and stores information and throws it back, in a subliminal way. It accepts everything as the truth: it influences thinking habits, speaking and acting with limited understanding.

There are positive ways in which we can work with our Subconscious Mind. The classic example is self-healing. We can be clever and use the gullibility of the Subconscious Mind to heal us. Whatever the subconscious believes, the body tends to manifest. If you are very ill, just start telling yourself that you are perfectly healthy. I guarantee you will heal quicker.

There are no limits to what you can achieve with positive thought; the possibilities are limitless. The key is to simply believe that what you are telling yourself will happen. Why shouldn't it? We are all simply bountiful and deserve everything we ask for; we are, after all, God incarnate.

But until we get rid of the fear and neurosis in the subconscious we will remain hindered and handicapped. As we go through life we begin to fill up the subconscious with fears, memories, hurts, pains and insecurities. Yet we actively tap in to the subconscious for answers, even though all it can do is regurgitate 'past' experiences. And we accept this totally, making us unable to move forwards. We remain stuck in the present because we are receiving information from the past. The subconscious believes that if something happened once before, then it will surely happen again. We may laugh at this situation, but it is the sad truth, and we fall for it every time.

You are what you think. If you think you are hurt, you will feel hurt. If you decide you do not hurt inside then the pain will not be there. It is just a question of choice. The minute you decide you do not want to be in pain, you simply will not be. It is that simple.

Another aspect of the Subconscious Mind is that it holds on to all our low self-esteem: all our so-called failures and defeats. It has accepted that all these negative emotions must be true, and it keeps telling us so. In addition, we, too, tend to believe all that we are told about ourselves.

So we have a choice: either we can start the cleaning-out process of the subconscious by seeing a therapist or we can start practising yoga and allow mantra and meditation to start dissolving false beliefs and free ourselves from their hold over us. It is just a case of one vibration absorbing the other. As we chant we create a vibration around and within us, as the issues from the subconscious come up, then the stronger, positive vibration from the mantra will absorb it. It is a very clear concept, and it absolutely works.

The Unconscious Mind

If we fail to clear out the subconscious, it will begin to overflow and then fall into our third and deepest level of the mind, the Unconscious Realm.

The Unconscious Mind is the vast arena that is not completely understood. All we know is that it is an extremely difficult part of the mind to reach and it is far more complicated to modify, let alone eliminate, behavioural patterns or neuroses. That is why it is so important to clear out the subconscious on a regular basis, to prevent overload into the unconscious. The best way is Sadhana (daily practice) and the very best methods are meditation and mantra.

Because Sadhana is a cleansing process, be prepared for the dust to fly. As you meditate, remain mindful that old feelings, fears and painful memories may come into your awareness. Remember that this is just confirmation that they are surfacing and can be eliminated. Just remain focused on the meditation while you observe your thoughts, without developing an attachment to them.

How to Tackle the Mind

There is a very powerful way to start the process of mastering the mind. It is the most positive way to apply the limitless potential and it is usually overlooked. This method is healing.

Healing has the ability to bring into wholeness those things that have been separated and lost in the individual. Healing brings all parts of us back together, restoring a sense of completeness and overwhelming joy as you contact aspects of yourself you felt you had 'lost'.

Living in today's modern world, we tend to believe that we are separate. These feelings of separation eat away at our psyche. When this feeling gets the better of us, we begin to experience comparison, judgement, resentment and anger. This leads to believing that we are not good enough; that someone else is better.

By being in a yoga class, or any group setting, you will begin to tackle the idea that you are separate. You are given the opportunity to join into this connectedness, to engage with other people on many levels. All those in a class will be there for a reason, even if the basic understanding of the reason is because you need to relax. Relax from what? As human beings, we long to be accepted and to engage with people at a much deeper level than our everyday lives allow us to.

When healing ourselves through yoga or meditation it will immediately have a very powerful effect on the mind. We start to release old beliefs that limit our full understanding of life. We will enter into a state of oneness, releasing the stuck energy that fixates on different parts of the body. When entering into the zone of healing many miracles start to occur.

When we actually stop and spend time with ourselves, the most amazing transformation occurs. I have witnessed this on countless occasions in yoga classes. There have been times when a person is suffering emotionally, but when the class is over they are beaming with happiness. To date, I have not taught a class where the participants have not hugged and talked afterwards. It is at that moment that the deepest truths come up and because you know you are in a safe and non-judgemental environment, you can speak your truth and let it go. It is truly miraculous. The freedom and release felt after sharing a part of yourself with a group is the greatest step forward anyone can achieve. Take your mind out of the constraints of your everyday affairs, connect with others and your own self-healing will be amplified many times over.

Mantra

A mantra can be a syllable, word or phrase in one of the sacred languages (such as Sanskrit and Gurbani) and sometimes in English, elevating or modifying consciousness through its meaning, the sound of the word, rhythm and tone.

Mantra is a very prominent part of Kundalini Yoga, as its results are immediate and powerful. *Mantra* means 'to vibrate the mind'; it is the projection of sound. Mantra comes under the umbrella of teaching known as 'Shabd Guru'. *Shabd* means 'that which cuts the ego', while *guru* is known as 'that which takes you from darkness to light'. It is often thought that the word *guru* means 'teacher'. A guru can be that, but the real understanding of the word is the journey itself, through the discovery of knowledge. A person can be the guru if they are the bearer of the knowledge, but only the knowledge that they impart is the key to transformation.

The ego is not a negative aspect of ourselves, but merely limiting and forgetful. When you act out of attachment to the ego, as if it was your real nature, then you will create pain, unhappiness and problems. Our true reality is beyond the ego; our true reality is abundant and has no boundaries.

In a cyclone you would go to the eye of the storm to escape its turbulent power. In an age that is swirling with chaotic change, we need to reach the centre of our storm; this is reached through the Neutral Mind, established to quell conscious and subconscious reactions to the ego. The Shabd Guru transforms you by removing the barriers erected by the needs of the ego.

By using mantras your consciousness will be raised to a level of a king and the angels will become your servants. Words are very potent. Everything you say becomes part of the Akashic Records and comes back to you. The Akashic Records are an energetic storehouse of every word, every deed, every action and reaction of all there ever has been. Everything that has ever happened has been energetically recorded, and this process will continue as long as there is life.

What you put out, you will get back, and that is a law of the Universe.

We can use mantras to neutralize thoughts, which is necessary in order to cleanse the subconscious mind of negativity.

Chanting a mantra is not singing, it is vibrating. By vibrating mantras, great quantities of energy are released into the body. This energy can be circulated in a variety of ways, until the body is immersed in a vast ocean of vibrating cosmic light. The secret is to vibrate the sound in the frontal cavities in the head. Also, it is very beneficial to vibrate in your chest; this is because the vibration will stimulate the Heart Centre. When you master this, you should start to vibrate the whole sound inside your body, which will cause waves of energy to travel through your whole being. Another important factor is to hear the mantra throughout your body. Try to get lost in the sound and surrender to its rhythm.

Why Do Mantras Work?

The science behind mantra is really quite simple. It is all to do with the movement of the tongue in the mouth, the use of language and the chemicals in the brain. There are no nerve connections between the sections of the brain. Messages are transmitted from one part to the other by fluids. Therefore, we have to work with these fluids to alter our consciousness and bring our personalities into harmony, to reflect who we truly are. The way we can alter this fluid is by our words, thoughts and our language. Our lips symbolize the Moon, or the feminine principle, and our tongue represents the Sun, or masculine principle. Speaking is an interplay between the two; a form of celestial intercourse.

There is no underestimating the power within mantras; it is a much-needed science for our time. Our patterns and behavioural traits are vibrations within us that have fallen out of alignment. We could never have been able to foresee this. As we accept that it is our character, we are not aware of the misalignment. For example, people often accept that they are an 'angry' person. 'That is just my personality', they tell you. No, it is not. That is their vibration. You can realign your personality to reflect the real essence of your Self.

It is surprising what a regular, daily 11-minute mantra can do for you, whether you aim to dissolve your anger, or some other misaligned vibration. Your inner Self will be at peace, you will radiate continuously with the vibration of the mantra, as every 24 hours you water the seed once again. It is an ancient secret that is now freely available; use this opportunity to try it.

The Science of Naad

Some of the mantras that we chant are in Gurbani, a language based on the science of the Naad, which is thousands of years old. All who would be king had to learn this valuable tool, which was written in liquid gold to preserve the teachings.

There are 84 meridian points located on the upper palate in the mouth. It is the tongue flicking the upper palate that causes the meridians to be stimulated. The rotation of the tongue stimulates certain parts of the hypothalamus. This, in turn, will cause the secretion of the pituitary and pineal glands, bringing about a change in the chemical composition in the brain. When the composition is enhanced with the components from these two glands, your personality, character and psyche will be transformed into a more balanced state.

The Meaning of Words

The Naad is in syllables, as a science. These syllables open up your 'naadis' (subtle nerves) throughout your body, therefore changing your chemistry. A person who speaks a positive word strengthens his physical body and his aura. When you speak negativity you will weaken yourself. It is destructive to utter anything against the Self or another person. Our happiness depends on continuous focusing on high, elevating thoughts.

Think of yourself as a Divine instrument with strings. When you pluck those strings all 30 trillion cells of the body vibrate. The vibration gives you shape, physically, emotionally and mentally.

You are created with 72 'surs', or wires. These each vary in dominance over a 72-hour period. The Crown Chakra has an impact on each of these strings or channels with a thousand-fold vibration, a wave of thoughts. Hence you have 72,000 movements, or vibratory impacts, which send energy through your system.

It is these 72,000 nerve endings that carry the vibration of the mantra to all parts of the body. When you chant you pick up an Infinite sound, a pattern that is timeless and vast, captured in a seed, in words. If the rhythm is right, your concentration focused and you allow yourself to surrender to its pulse, then the central nervous system vibrates it and you simply listen.

When we chant, it is a vibration direct to the Infinite Mind – God.

All our thoughts in the mind are vibratory frequencies: happiness, sorrow, joy or regret. These thought waves determine the programme our mind 'plays'. Which one we decide to act on will become our vibration and this is what we project to others. We can choose what we choose to be at any time.

When we chant we choose to invoke the positive power contained in those syllables. The sound current can cut through almost any negativity in the psyche. It does not matter whether we understand the meaning of the words or not. We are creating, with every word that we speak and every thought that we think. Every vibration that we send out will come back to us.

The Universe is the Uni-Verse, we are all one sound.

Ways to Practise

You can choose a mantra by looking in the Meditations and Sadhana chapters in this book (*see pages 173 and 74*). Here are a few guidelines to follow:

1. Turn the phone off and invoke a feeling of peace in your personal space. Perhaps light a candle or burn some incense.
2. Always tune in with Ong Namo Guru Dev Namo *(see page 98)*; even if you are only going to do a meditation. This will link you to the Golden Chain, an energetic thread to all the masters. To understand the full process of getting ready for either a kriya or a meditation, please see the section on Tuning In in Part 2 *(see page 97)*.
3. Remember to vibrate the mantra, not sing it.
4. Keep your spine straight and your eyes closed.
5. Chant from your Navel Point for maximum power.
6. Be aware of your tongue on the meridian points.
7. All mantras should be practised for the designated times.
8. Always practise in the most peaceful part of your home, and always return to that spot, so that the energy can build up there. When you next sit down, the energy will take you deeper into meditation, as you will be building an energetic space, a haven to retreat to.
9. When you have finished, inhale deeply and allow the energy to circulate throughout your body. Even though you have stopped chanting you should still hear the sound current swirling around you.
10. When you are ready to move away from your space, finish by chanting Sat Nam at least three times, sealing your practice with the affirmation that 'I am the embodiment of truth'.

Pronunciation Guide

a	as in spa or baa
ai	as in rye or wry
an	as in can or tan
ar	as in car or jar
ay	as in day or play
ee	as in reed or seed
o	as in so or go
ong	as in song or gong
sat	as in but or nut
u	as in through or hue

> Do the best you can, and let God do the rest.

Pranayama

The breath is a fundamental tool for the student of kundalini. Mastery of the breath is the foundation for the ability to open the range of your emotions, to control your moods, promote health and develop concentration.

To begin with we need to understand what breath is. For the yogi it is the combination of the physical breath and the subtle life force of the body and mind, known as Prana. Consider the breath and its movement as being connected to all your thoughts and your emotions. See the breath as a wave or a current that flows in and out. Become aware of the intimate relationship between the breath and the words you speak. When you breathe slowly and deeply, your words will become gentle and there will be less need for mindless chatter; instead your words will hold strength and grace. Your words will hold the truth of who you are. When the breath is quick, so too will be your speech. You may say things that you will later regret; you will be speaking from erratic thoughts. In the chapter on the mind (*see page* 46), we spoke of how the mind follows the breath; when we slow the breath the mind will follow immediately. It is also the same for speech. We slow the breath, we calm the mind and the words will become truthful reflections of our true Selves.

When we speak our truth, our relationships will begin to harmonize. As you reveal your truth you, in turn, will allow others to do the same.

Look at the diagram below. The lower chakras represent the impulses and the animal nature in us. They are necessary and full of vitality. When your words come from this realm they are ordinary, everyday speech. The breath pulses with feelings and calls on certain words to express them. The Heart Centre is where we are balanced as human beings. The upper chakras are where we are merged into the subtle realms and it is in the Eighth Chakra where we are merged in transcendent liberation. What we need to do is to pull the two triangles together and merge at the Heart Centre. When this happens our word will be true and soft. We will be speaking with wholeness. As yogis we must learn to let go of the idea that breath is respiration. Give your breath the importance it has to shape your life. If you learn to regulate it with reverence and precision you will always have resources and spirit at your command.

Long, Deep Breathing

How much breath we take in is a reflection of how full of energy we will feel. Within breath there is life force. The deeper we breathe the more life force will we consume. If you always feel tired or have no get-up-and-go, spend three minutes every morning doing long, deep breathing. But since our normal everyday breathing is automatic, we need to cultivate our breath to become deeper. It is the subtle aspect of Prana within the breath that energizes the body and mind. The quantity, quality and circulation of each breath creates the foundation of a vital and creative life.

How to do it

First we need to distinguish the three parts of the breath; the abdominal, the thoracic and the clavicular. A full breath starts deep in the abdomen, expanding the belly, then expanding the chest and finally lifting the upper ribs and clavicle. The exhale is the reverse, the upper deflates, followed by the chest and then as the abdomen empties so we pull back on the navel towards the spine.

Abdominal breath

Come into a sitting position (Easy Pose) on the floor or chair, with the soles of your feet on the floor (*see page* 105). Allow your hands to fall into your lap. Be very relaxed, and allow the breath to be at a normal pace. Bring your attention to your navel and begin to take a slow, deep breaths in through your nostrils. Expand your belly and allow it to move forwards. Then exhale and pull your navel back towards your spine, to completely empty the abdomen.

Try this a few times, until you feel the opening of your abdomen. If you have difficulties, place your hands on your belly and try, with the breath, to push your belly forwards against your hands and then pull it back with the exhale, deep inside your torso. Continue for a minute.

Chest breath

Inhale slowly, using only your chest muscles between the ribs. Focus on this part of your body

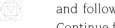

and follow the sensation of expansion. Exhale completely, but do not use your abdomen. Continue for a minute.

Clavicular breath

Contract the navel and keep your abdomen tight. Lift your chest without inhaling. Now inhale slowly by expanding your shoulders and your collarbone. Exhale as you keep your chest lifted. Continue for a minute.

When all three are combined, you will have experienced a long, deep breath.

How to do Long, Deep Breathing

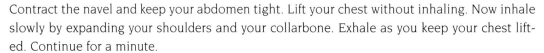

Sit straight. Begin with the inhale, with an abdominal breath. Then add the chest breath and finish with the clavicular breath. Do all three in a smooth motion, flowing from one to the other. As you exhale start by relaxing the clavicle and then slowly emptying the chest. Finally pull in the navel to force out any remaining breath. Continue in a rhythmic way for as long as the exercise states.

The benefits
- relaxing and calming
- gives you clarity and patience
- reduces and prevents build-up of toxins in the lungs
- stimulates the brain chemicals that help to fight depression
- restores the aura
- builds alertness and formulates good decision-making
- pumps the spinal fluid to the brain
- expands your lungs
- cleanses the blood
- activates and cleanses nerve channels
- aids speeding up healing within the Emotional and Physical Bodies
- reduces insecurity and fear

o feeds your electromagnetic field, which will make you less likely to fall victim to accidents, sickness and negativity.

Breath of Fire

This breath is unique to Kundalini Yoga. It is used to accompany many postures and exercise sets. This breath needs to be mastered so that it becomes automatic and accurate.

How to do it

Sit in a comfortable sitting posture such as Easy Pose (*see page* 105), or on a chair. The breath is rapid, rhythmic and continuous. It is equal on the inhale and exhale. It is mostly the dead air space that is vibrated in and out of the lungs. Breath of Fire is powered by the Navel Point and solar plexus. The chest stays relaxed and slightly lifted. It is always practised through the nostrils, unless otherwise stated. The focus is on the inhale and the exhale being equal. The breath is rapid, deep and powerful, with the breath sounding like a sniff. The rhythm is two or three breaths per second. At first do not try to go fast. It is better to begin to practise at a slower rate. To understand the importance of the navel movement you could place your hands on your belly to feel it jump back and forth. In the initial stages it is very helpful to experience the breath while lying on your back, with your hands on your belly. The exhale is similar to when you blow your nose: fast and powerful as you pull your Navel Point back towards your spine.

Begin to practise for one to three minutes. You should not experience any dizziness or lightheadedness, which indicates hyperventilation. Tests have measured both the brain waves and blood chemistry for Breath of Fire and it has shown that it is not hyperventilation. Tingling and energetic sensations are completely normal as your body adjusts to the new breath and new stimulation of your nerves. If you concentrate at your Brow Point, this feeling will quickly pass.

Remember to keep the spine straight, with your eyes closed but held at the Brow Point. Persevere, as it does take a little practice. There have been reports stating a reduction in addictive impulses.

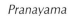

The benefits
- releases old toxins from the lungs and blood vessels
- expands lung capacity
- reduces addictive impulses for drugs, smoking and unhealthy foods
- strengthens the nervous system
- increases physical endurance
- energizes the blood, which aids healing
- creates a focused and neutral state of mind
- boosts the immune system and helps prevent diseases
- promotes synchronization of the biorhythms in different parts of the body
- energizes the whole mind and body

Holding the Breath

Fundamental to mastering the breath is the ability to hold the breath in or out. This is one of the first skills that we need to learn. Because it is so elementary it can be poorly performed since it has been least studied. After every posture and meditation you either hold the breath in or out.

Many people, when holding the breath, push the chin out, tighten the neck and stiffen the tongue. This is not correct as it creates a great pressure in the eyes, heart, neck and the back of the skull.

The correct way to hold the breath in or out is to suspend it. To suspend the breath means to relax the muscles of the diaphragm, ribs and abdomen. Everything should be relaxed. Only the breath is held in suspension.

When holding the breath it is important to maintain a straight spine, with your chin tucked in to lengthen the back of the neck.

Holding the Breath In

Sit straight, with your chin tucked in to lengthen the back of the neck. Keep your eyes closed, inhale deeply and suspend the breath. You will reach a point when the brain tells you to exhale. Instead, try inhaling a tiny bit more and then exhale slowly. Keep checking that your body is relaxed.

Holding the Breath Out

Sit straight, with your chin tucked in to lengthen the back of your neck. Keep your eyes closed, exhale deeply to begin, and then inhale deeply and exhale as you pull your Navel Point back towards the spine. Lift your lower chest and diaphragm. Become still and calm. Again you will feel the urge to inhale, but instead exhale a little more. This can extend the suspension significantly, without any strain or struggle.

The goal is to switch the metabolic activity, achieve nervous system balance and gain emotional control. If you begin to experience dizziness or disorientation, stop. Dizziness is not enlightenment. The goal is a gradual reconditioning of the nervous system. You must build this practice with regularity and patience.

Throughout the practice observe the changes taking place in the body and mind. Breath suspension will make your body work at a higher level of efficiency. It will also train you to use good judgement under pressure. Breath-retention is a powerful tool for creating psychic heat. It is often used to stimulate kundalini arousal. Follow directions carefully.

Alternative Nostril Breathing

The nostrils are the gateways to the Pranic Body, through which the Prana comes into your body. The right nostril accesses the Pingala, while the left accesses the Ida.

Sit with a straight spine in Easy Pose, with the Neck Lock applied (*see Bandhs, page* 70). Using your right hand, place your right thumb over your right nostril and inhale slowly through the left nostril. Place your right ring finger over your left nostril and exhale slowly through your right nostril. Continue this practice for the stated time. You can try this practice for various lengths of time, from three to 11, to 31 minutes. Breathing through the left nostril is calming and tranquillizing, while through the right the effect is energizing and action-oriented. By combining the two you are stimulating both, and creating balance within the main energetic pathway in the body. This practice can revitalize your whole nervous system, and is particularly helpful if you are feeling 'off-centre'.

Left-Nostril Breathing

If you are feeling stressed, angry, agitated and anxious apply left-hand nostril breathing for five minutes, to completely calm down. Left-nostril breathing is a great technique if you are having trouble sleeping or when you need to relax.

Sit with your spine straight. Using the thumb of your right hand, keeping your fingers together and pointing straight up close your right nostril. Begin long, deep breathing through your left nostril. Twenty-six long, deep breaths will bring you completely to peace and calm. In Kundalini Yoga we often repeat things for 26 times, as two plus six equals eight. Eight is associated with the number for Infinity, God. When using the number eight in Kundalini Yoga we are tapping in to the source of Infinity and reproducing its energy within us in the Earth Realm.

Right-Nostril Breathing

Right-nostril breathing is great when you are exhausted, yet know you have to keep going. It is good to practise it when you get your mid-afternoon slump at work.

Start the practice as above, but using your left thumb to block your left nostril. Again 26 breaths will increase your energy and you will feel revitalized.

Sitali Pranayama

This is done by breathing in through the mouth with a curled tongue, and exhaling through the nose, but with your tongue still protruding through your mouth. This practice cools the body and lowers fever. It is also very beneficial as an aid to giving up smoking. Practise the breath when you get the urge to have a cigarette. The addictive impulse will diminish if you practise the breath the instant you get the urge. Daily practice is a prescription for good health. You will notice after the practice that the tongue may taste coppery or metallic. This is normal, as toxins are being lifted up and out of the body. Continue for at least three minutes, working towards 31 maximum.

Sit in Easy Pose with your hands in Gyan Mudra or in your lap. With a straight spine, stick out and curl your tongue into a 'U' shape. Slowly begin to breathe in through your mouth, and then exhale slowly through your nose. Continue to breathe in this pattern for at least three minutes, working towards 31 minutes.

Whistle Breath

Sit in Easy Pose (*see page* 105) with a straight spine, with the hands in Gyan Mudra (*see page* 67) or in your lap. Begin to inhale and exhale through a puckered 'O' mouth to create a whistle sound on both the inhale and the exhale. This has a profound effect on your consciousness. In a group setting the sound is wonderful and very powerful. Continue for three minutes, working towards 31 maximum.

Mudras and Bandhs

The central aim of the physical efforts of yoga is to generate a special capacity and flow of life force within the body and the aura. This energy is increased in both quantity and quality. It is then directed into a natural pattern of circulation that releases the healing powers of the body and the discriminative functions of the mind. In this state of inner health and clarity the individual's life will start to expand in all directions. Kundalini Yoga benefits the body but also uses it as a vehicle for enhanced consciousness. The energy that flows into the body is called Prana, while the outgoing energy is called Apana. They are the two aspects of the life-force energy.

Mudras

These are hand positions that lock and guide the energy flow to the brain. By curling, crossing, stretching and touching certain parts of the fingers and palms we can invoke and project certain energies and guide them to different parts of the brain. Every mudra works with the elements. Using the hands in this way can allow us effectively to talk to the Subtle, Mental and Physical Bodies.

The hand is magical as well as functional. The hand expresses our moods in each minute gesture. If you look at your palm you will see that the lines form intriguing patterns. If you can understand the coding, your hands reveal an energy map of your consciousness and health. The yogis mapped out the hand areas and their associated reflexes to a certain part of the body and brain. Each finger relates to a certain tattva (element) of which all life is formed, and represents the five sections of the brain. Each area also reflects different emotions or behaviours. Each mudra listed below is a technique for giving clear messages to the mind-body energy system. In most kriyas and meditations the mudras are performed with both hands, unless otherwise stated.

The mudras are sometimes performed reversed for men and women because of the differences of polarity within our energy.

Gyan Mudra

Place the tip of your index finger against your thumb tip. This stimulates your knowledge and ability. The energy of the index finger is often symbolized by Jupiter, the planet representing expansion. This mudra is the most commonly used. It gives you receptivity, knowledge and calmness.

When you bend your index finger under your thumb pad, the fingernail is under the second joint of the thumb. This then becomes the 'active' form of Gyan Mudra, as shown. This is usually used with a powerful pranayama or meditation. This practice amplifies the power of the mudra, and gives a short and direct route to the mind-body computer.

Shuni Mudra

Place the tip of your middle finger against your thumb tip. This mudra is said to give patience and discernment. The middle finger is often symbolized by the planet Saturn. Saturn represents the taskmaster, the law of Karma, responsibility and courage to deliver what is asked of you.

Surya Mudra

Place the tip of your ring finger against the thumb tip. Practising it gives you revitalizing energy, nervous strength and good health. The quality of the ring finger is symbolized by the Sun. The Sun represents energy, health and sexuality.

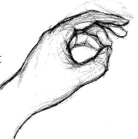

Buddhi Mudra

Place the tip of your little finger against your thumb tip. This mudra opens up the capacity to communicate clearly and intuitively. It also stimulates psychic development. The little finger is symbolized by Mercury as quickness and the mental powers of communication.

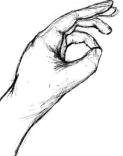

Venus Lock

This lock gets its name because it connects the positive and negative sides of the venus mound on each hand to the thumbs. The venus mound is the fleshy area at the base of the thumb and the thumbs represent the ego. It is symbolized by the planet Venus, associated with the energy of sensuality and sexuality. The mudra balances the sexual energy and promotes glandular balance. It also enhances the ability to concentrate easily if you bring the mudra down on to your lap while adopting a meditative posture.

To form the mudra place your palms opposite each other and interlace your fingers with the right little finger at the bottom. Place your right thumb tip in the webbed part of your left hand, between the thumb and index finger. The left thumb tip presses against the fleshy mound of the base of the right thumb. The mudra position is reversed for men.

Prayer Mudra

Place your palms together in a 'prayer position'. The fingers and thumbs need to line up and connect with the opposite palm. The positive side of the body (the right, male side) and the negative (left, female side) are neutralized. This mudra balances out the opposing energies within the individual. This mudra is always used when initially centring yourself in preparation for doing a kriya.

Bear Grip

Place your left palm facing out from your chest with the thumb down. Place the palm of your right hand facing your chest. Curl the fingers together to form two fists gripping each other. This mudra stimulates the heart and intensifies concentration.

Buddha Mudra

Place your left hand on top of your right. There must be no gaps between the fingers and you need to form a small cup in your palms. The position is very gentle yet focused. The palms should be face up in your lap while you are in a meditative pose. The thumb tips also need to be touching, forming a small triangle away from the palms. The right palm needs to rest on top of the left for men.

In all these mudras exert enough pressure to feel the flow of energy through the 'nadis' (psychic channels) up into your arms. Make sure you do not exert too much pressure, whitening the fingertips.

Bandhs

The bandhs are the locks applied to certain parts of the body to mix and hold the Prana and Apana, so that these two energies can blend and then be distributed throughout the body and mind.

The bandhs are usually applied after an exercise, or sometimes the lock is held throughout the whole posture. The locks can be held on the in-breath or the out-breath, but instruction must always be followed as to which breath it should be. This application has enormous impact on the entire body–mind system.

There are three main bandhs: Jalandhara Bandh (Neck Lock), Uddiyana Bandh (Diaphragm Lock) and Mul Bandh (Root Lock). When all three locks are applied together it is called Maha Bandh, or the Great Lock.

These techniques are well recorded in the classic sources of yoga practice such as the hatha yoga, Pradipika, and the tantric exposition of the Sage Gheranda, in Gheranda Samhita.

It is a fundamental law that at the end of most exercises in Kundalini Yoga that you will apply the Mul Bandh, though it is not asked for in detail in all instances. You will be told to put yourself into a certain posture, with a sound current and breathing pattern. But all the kriyas have certain things that are assumed. First is the proper posture and the second is the locks.

YOGI BHAJAN

Neck Lock, or Jalandhara Bandh

This is the first and most commonly applied of the locks. It is a general rule to apply it in all chanting meditations and during most pranayama exercises. Whenever you are holding the breath in or out it is usually applied unless stated otherwise.

To apply the lock, sit comfortably, with your spine straight. Lift your chest and sternum up. At the same time gently stretch the back of your neck straight by pulling the chin inwards. Your chin and the chest move towards each other so that your chin rests in the notch of the collarbone at the top of your breastbone.

Your head stays level and the muscles of your neck and throat remain loose. Do not force your head forwards or down. Relax the muscles of the face and brow and keep your head centred without tilting from side to side. The idea is to seal the energy that is generated in the upper areas of the brain stem.

This bandh does several things at once. It opens the channel between the torso and the head, so that the energy can freely flow to wherever it needs to go, according to the technology of the kriya. It prevents undue changes in blood pressure that can sometimes be induced by exercise and breathing. It acts as a safety valve that regulates that pressure and gets rid of any dizziness. It stimulates and balances the thyroid and parathyroid glands. It directs the flow of Pranic energy into the central channel past the neck and into the central channel relative to the heart. When the lock is applied the heart is calmed and the flow of energy becomes natural. The word *jala* refers to the brain and its watery secretions; and *dhara* means 'the upward pull' or 'open gate'. Jalandhara is the upward pull that opens the gate to the brain's watery nectars. By applying this lock there is an increased concentration of those secretions from the pituitary, pineal and hypothalamus glands that allow a new level of connection between them.

Diaphragm Lock, or Uddiyana Bandh

The name of this lock, Uddiyana, comes from the Sanskrit 'to fly up'. This refers to the effect of the energy in the lower abdomen. There is a great barrier formed by the diaphragm between the thorax and the lower abdomen. It is a physical muscular barrier as well as an energetic one. This lock crosses that barrier. The functions below the barrier are more unconscious, instinctual and reactive, while the functions above are more conscious, flexible and refined. For greater understanding of this, please see the chapter on chakras (*see page* 82).

To apply Uddiyana Bandh sit comfortably, with a straight spine. Inhale deeply and completely exhale the breath. Pull your entire abdominal region, especially above the Navel Point back towards the spine and upwards. Lift your chest, but never apply this lock and collapse the chest downwards. Gently press the lower thoracic and lumbar spine forwards. Keep the lift strongly applied for a period of 10–60 seconds, according to your endurance. Hold it in an inner mood of equilibrium and calm. Then release the lock by relaxing the abdomen and gradually inhaling. Do not release the Neck Lock while you are doing this and never do it on a full stomach. Only apply this lock on the exhale.

To learn this well you can practise it in a standing position. Stand straight, with your feet a shoulder-width apart. Bend forwards slightly, with your hands on your knees. Lift your chest slightly, inhale and then exhale and apply the lock.

You may well feel slight heat in your ear lobes or neck; this is the sensation of the energy rising and is perfectly normal.

This lock is associated with youthfulness and the slowing of all degenerative ageing. It is a stimulant for cleansing as in either position the intestines and the heart will receive a direct internal massage.

The Uddiyana Bandh helps to enhance the energies from the solar centre at the solar plexus. This is the centre for the element of fire. As you pull the lock back the fire is strengthened and the Heart Chakra is opened. Kindness, compassion and patience will become an inherent quality with regular practice of this lock.

Root Lock, or Mul Bandh

This is the most complex of the three body locks. It is like a hydraulic lock at the base of the spine. The word 'mul' is the root, base or source. It co-ordinates, blends and stimulates the energies involved with the rectum, sex organs and Navel Point. It redirects excess sexual energy into creativity and bodily repair. Ninety per cent of sexual energy is used to fuel the immune system. If there is a lack of sexual vitality this lock will enhance it. This bandh is frequently applied at the end of an exercise or an exercise series to crystallize its effects. It is usually applied with Jalandhara Bandh.

Mul Bandh is a smooth motion that consists of three parts. The first part is the contraction of the anus. You squeeze the anus shut and then lift the anal sphincter upwards. Then you contract the area around the sex organs. This is experienced as a slight lift and inward pull of the pubic bone. It is a bit like stopping the flow of urine. Then contract the lower abdomen and Navel Point back towards the spine. These three actions applied together in a smooth, rapid, flowing movement is the Mul Bandh. This lock can be applied with the breath held in or out. This lock is pulled with the area above the navel relaxed.

The Root Lock performs several functions. The key function is the blending of the Prana and Apana at the Navel Centre. The Root Lock redirects the flow of Apana from its normal downwards course towards the First Chakra. When the lock is applied the energy is blocked and has no choice but to go upwards towards the Navel Centre to join the Pranic energy. When these two energies meet an inner heat or 'tapa' is created, which then opens the entrance to the Sushmana, the central channel of energy up the spine. This bandh starts the process of transformation from the gross to the subtle.

The Great Lock, or Maha Bandh

The Great Lock is the application of all three locks simultaneously, while the breath is held out. The practice and perfection of this lock is said to cure many ailments such as high or low blood pressure, poor circulation and excessive preoccupation with sexual fantasy. With the three locks applied the body is in a perfect healing state. The glandular and nervous systems become revitalized and rejuvenated.

This lock is performed in various postures and combined with different mudras. However, to practise these locks it is always easier to perform them in Easy Pose or in a comfortable sitting position. I recommend that you practise the Root Lock first, working towards the Diaphragm Lock, the Neck Lock and then finally mastering the Great Lock. This lock is part of the central infrastructure of Kundalini Yoga.

Sadhana

Sadhana is, simply, daily spiritual practice. It is three things: a commitment, a discipline and a devotion. It is a commitment to the Higher Self; it is a discipline to the mind and its devotion to the Creator, who created you.

All serious forms of self-discovery will include Sadhana within their teachings because it deals with the very thing that keeps us from liberation, the ego. It is a method to achieve self-victory. Yogic scriptures require that we give one-tenth of our day to Sadhana, that is two and a half hours. The specified time for Sadhana is in the ambrosial hours between 4 and 7am. This is when the element of ether is prominent. This is the time that the auric protection and guidance of the teacher is the most prevalent. In these hours the Prana is most concentrated, as few people are awake. The clutter and noise of everyone going about their business will not be there to interfere with what you are doing. The element of ether is also known as the astral light. The astral realm is around us at all times; it is a reality living alongside our reality, a dimension within our own dimension. We rarely even stop to recognize this, let alone be with it and understand it. This is the realm of thoughts, emotions and ideas; it is subtle stimulation. Doing Sadhana at this time of the day will bring very positive results.

To really get to grips with making major changes in your life and within yourself, do Sadhana. That is the secret of all secrets, within all forms of self-liberation. It is such a simple act, but it takes commitment, discipline and devotion.

When I was first told about Sadhana, especially the time of day it would take place, I groaned and told myself I could never do it. But during the time I was training to become a teacher I had no choice. I now had to face my biggest challenge. Getting up at 4.30am was not actually too bad. Having a cold shower was fun, and preparing myself physically for Sadhana felt very sacred, as though I was performing a ritual. Coming together with a group to practise Sadhana was wonderful. I knew the moment I entered that room, I had achieved Sadhana, I had done it, and I was a success. 100 per cent success is getting to Sadhana. We started at 5am and finished at 7.30am. By the time we had finished I felt so alive, so full of life and so ready to get on with the day. Sadhana is a powerful process; it takes all you have got to get there and it takes even more to stay focused and alert for the duration. But what I have come to realize is that the barriers we have to break down in order to actually do it, is the binding of the ego that we must learn to master.

Initially, Sadhana does not have to last two and a half hours. It can be as little as 11 minutes, done every morning at the same time, ideally in the same place. I suggest that you just do a little every day. I cannot emphasize enough the importance of setting your own energy daily; you will grow at such an abundant rate. When I do not do Sadhana my old patterns start to return, I begin to lose my connection to God, I begin to feel lost again and then the suffering starts to come back. I absolutely believe in this practice, so please find out if this is true for you. If it is, then this knowledge will be one of the greatest gifts you will ever receive.

Sadhana is a deep, cleansing process from this lifetime and many more that have gone before. It is a very powerful clearing of the subconscious, which pushes and pulls at us. To be in happiness and joy we must tackle the purification within that aspect of us. When we work on the subconscious mind, you may find the most ugly and unpleasant thoughts surfacing. You may even feel anger, rage, annoyance and frustration. That is a positive sign that you are plunging into the depths of negativity that are within all of us. I have been quite peaceful in Sadhana, when the vilest thought has unexpectedly crossed my mind. I was shocked that I could think such a thing. On other occasions, I have been so enraged in my personal practice that I have screamed out in anger. If you too experience such unexpected emotions, go through them; continue even if you are in floods of tears, for the gates of liberation are just around the corner.

Preparation

You can do Sadhana by yourself or in a group. Being in a group will amplify the energy, plus it will give you more of an incentive to actually get up and get there.

The place where you do your Sadhana should be clean, quiet and have a feel of being a 'special place'. Keep this place sacred. This is your space.

Sadhana actually begins the night before; you will need to get an early night if it is your first time. Say to yourself as you go to sleep 'I will get up, I will get up'. Try to do your Sadhana at the same time every day, as the energy will begin to build in the space. You will be creating a vortex of very positive and powerful healing energy. Even going to that space just to sit for a few moments will fill you with powerful healing and peaceful light.

When you first get up you will need to cleanse your body, and the very best way is with a cold shower. Having a cold shower will awaken the body and mind from their sleeping patterns. The circulation will be boosted as the capillaries become stimulated as well as the nervous system being strengthened.

After the shower, rub some almond oil into your skin. This is a valuable yogic practice that keeps your skin youthful. Next put on some clean, comfortable, natural clothes, preferably white in colour. Wearing white truly expands the aura. You will need a shawl or blanket during the practice. Again this should be made of natural fabrics: wool, silk or cotton. Keep these clothes just for the practice of yoga and Sadhana, as over time these garments will absorb the vibrations of the practice. Just by putting them on you will instantly become in tune.

Next you will need something to sit on. This can either be a wool or cotton blanket or a sheepskin. In ancient times many yogis practised on animal skins, the beginners used sheepskins, progressing to deerskins and eventually the master would have a tiger skin. The reason we choose something natural to sit on insulates our psycho-electromagnetic field.

Light a candle and burn some incense just to give your mind stimulation that you are about to be engaged in something very special. At all times keep your spine straight. When you are ready tune in with the Adi Mantra (*see How to Begin, page* 97). The minute you chant this mantra you will be filled with an inflow of energy and light coming in to your mind and body.

Sadhana should include physical exercise, meditation, mantra and prayer. Ideally you should choose quite a strong exercise set, to remove any blocks and tensions in the body after sleeping. Take the time to meditate after every exercise, just for a minute or so, to observe the energy and the mind. Another very important part of Sadhana is mantra. Yogi Bhajan has given us a Sadhana to do until the year 2013. This includes all the elements of a good and well-rounded Sadhana.

After you have finished chanting the mantra, carry on listening and meditate on the sound. The sound current will be all around you, vibrating in the ether. Allow yourself to listen as this powerful technique can take you out of body consciousness and into bliss.

After Sadhana you will need to relax for 10 to 20 minutes. You need to allow time for the mind and body to process the energy you have raised and then fall back into equilibrium. During this time, it is fine to sleep; you may find that you have out-of-body experiences or vivid dreams. The very best position to relax in is Corpse Pose, which is lying on your back with your palms face up, legs slightly open, with your ankles flopped to the sides. Your eyes are closed, with a real sense of surrender within the body and mind. It is at this time that you cover yourself with your shawl or blanket. Just let go.

When you come round, you should finish with a prayer. The Universe is really listening, and this is only because it is at this time that you will be truly projecting with the depths of your being. The Universe is always listening, but it takes a bit of work to pray with the whole of your Self. Remember, when you pray you can ask for anything. We need to drop the guilt about asking for something for ourselves. The best way to pray is to open your heart and be grateful for being able to pray with such devotion. For it is only we humans that can do such a thing. Yogi Bhajan has advised that we inhale, hold the breath, pray and then exhale. Keep going like this until you are finished.

Always end Sadhana with the closing sequence (*see* How to Begin, *page* 102).

Sadhana should include:
1. Yoga
2. Meditation
3. Mantra
4. Prayer

If you have this book in your hands, you may as well take the gift that is being offered to you. Lose the obsession with time, as every moment that passes is an opportunity for further discovery. May God be with you.

Yogi Bhajan's Morning Sadhana for the Aquarian Age

Throughout the years Yogi Bhajan has periodically adjusted the content of the morning Sadhana. He gave the following sequence of mantras on 21 June 1992, with instructions to continue chanting them in this order for the next 21 years, until 2013. There is no gap or pause between the different mantra sections. Total time is 62 minutes. It is strongly recommended that you buy a Sadhana tape or CD (*see page* 231) to experience the correct rhythm and tone of the mantras.

1. Ek Ong Kar Sat Nam Siri Wahe Guru (7 minutes)
   One Creator created this creation. Truth is His name. Great beyond description is His infinite wisdom
   - sit with a straight spine
   - apply the Neck Lock
   - deeply inhale and chant Ek Ong Kar
   - inhale again and chant Sat Nam until you are out of breath, then whisper Siri, which is brief
   - then, inhale a half breath and chant Wahe Guru
   - inhale deeply to continue repeating the cycle

* This mantra is known as Long Ek Ong Kar (Morning Call) it is highly recommended that you purchase a Sadhana CD or tape (*see page* 231), as this mantra has a very precise rhythm and tone in its practice.

2. Waah Yantee Kar Yantee (7 minutes)
   Waah Yantee, Kar Yantee, Jag Doot Patee, Aadak It Waahaa, Brahmaadeh Traysha Guru, It Waahe Guru Great Macroself, Creative Self, All that is Creative through time. All that

is the Great One. Three aspects of God: Brahma, Vishnu, Mahesh. That is Wahe Guru.

3. The Mool Mantra (7 minutes)
   The Mool (root) mantra lets you experience the depth and consciousness of your soul.
   a) IMPORTANT: leave a slight 'space' between ajoonee and saibhang. Do not run the words together.
   b) Emphasize and slightly extend the 'ch' sound at the end of the word sach. This adds power.

Ek Ong Kar	One Creator, Creation
Sat Nam	Truth Named
Kartaa Purakh	Doer of Everything
Nirbhao	Fearless
Nirvair	Revengeless
Akaal Moorat	Undying
Ajoonee	Unborn
Saibhang	Self-illumined, Self-existent
Gur Prasaad	Guru's Grace
Jap	repeat
Aad Sach	True in the Beginning
Jugaad Sach	True throughout the Ages
Hai Bhee Sach	True even now
Naanak Hosee Bhee Sach	Nanak says Truth shall ever be

This mantra gives you the capacity to retain rulership. There are 108 elements in the universe and 108 letters in this mantra (in the original Gurmukhi script).

4. Sat Siri, Siri Akal (7 minutes)
The Mantra for the Aquarian Age'

Sat Siri	Great Truth
Siri Akaal	Great Undying
Siri Akall	Great Undying
Maha Akaal	Great Deathless
Maha Akaal	Great Deathless
Sat Nam	Truth is His Name
Akaal Moorat	Deathless image of God
Wahe Guru	Great beyond description is His Wisdom

5. Rakhe Rakhan Har (7 minutes)

This is a sound current of protection against all negative forces that move against one's walk on the path of destiny, both inner and outer. It cuts like a sword through every opposing vibration, thought, word and action.

Rakhay rakhanahaar aap ubaaria-an
Gur kee pairee paa-ay kaaj savaari-an
Hoaa aap day-aal manaho na visaari-an
Saadh janaa kai sang bhavajal taari-an
Saakat nindak dusht khin maa-eh bidaari-an
Tis saahib kee tayk Naanak manai maa-eh
Jis simrat sukh ho-ay sagalay dookh jaa-eh

Thou who savest, save us all and take us across
Uplifting and giving the excellence
You gave us the touch of the lotus fee of the
Guru, and all our jobs are done.
You have become merciful, kind and

Compassionate; and so our mind does
not forget Thee.

In the company of the holy beings you take us
From misfortunes and calamities, scandals,
And disrepute
Godless, slanderous enemies – you finish
them in Timelessness
That great Lord is my anchor
Nanak, keep Him firm in your mind.
By meditating and repeating his Name.
All happiness comes and all sorrows and pain go away.

6. Wahe Guru Wahe Jio (22 minutes)
   To be most effective, chant this mantra sitting in Hero Pose: Sit on your left heel, keep your spine straight, with your right knee against your chest, and your hands in Prayer Pose at your breastbone. Your eyes are focused at the tip of your nose.

   Wahe Guru, Wahe Guru, Wahe Guru, Wahe Jio

   Wahe Guru is a mantra of ecstasy. There is no real translation of it. Jio, is an affection ate but still respectful variation of the word Jee, which means Soul.

7. Guru Ram Das Guru (5 minutes)
   Guru Guru Wahe Guru Guru Ram Das Guru

   These syllables are in praise of the consciousness of Guru Ram Das and invoke his spiritual light, guidance and protective grace.

Chakras

Chakra is a Sanskrit word meaning 'wheel'. Like a wheel a chakra can spin slowly or rapidly. Our chakras spin in relation to the degree of energy in the system. They are to be found in every one of us. Just as everyone has a Physical Body, so too do we have a Subtle Body. These chakras serve as a bridge between the physical matter and the subtle matter.

There is much information freely available on chakras, and the subject is well worth researching. But please take what you read with a pinch of salt, as only your experience will give you a true understanding.

I have decided to map out a simple understanding of the eight major chakras in the body and how they may affect you. Since teaching Kundalini Yoga I have noticed how fascinated many people become with the chakra system, and how easy it is for beginners to fully learn about their subtle anatomy. I have illustrated the symbols of the chakras being worked on in the sections on the yoga kriyas and meditations (*see pages* 117 *and* 171). This will give you a greater understanding about what you are working on when you practise a particular posture or meditation. I have found this works very well for identifying what stage you have arrived at within the dynamics of your three-fold structure (body, mind, spirit).

As you begin to understand the chakras, so your awareness will begin to expand. You will then be able to identify where your consciousness is and have the tools readily available to work through that particular area, should a block arise.

The chakras themselves are part of a greater network of subtle energies. The function of the chakras is to convey the life force to the nucleus of every cell in the body. We cannot study subtle anatomy within, relating it to our physical anatomy, as it is the chakras that facilitate the flow and interchange of energies between the subtle and the physical. The development of Kirlian photography has now revealed the reality of life-force energy for the first time. It is now possible to see the energy emanations in a photographic form.

There are three principal channels through which this Pranic energy flows. These channels are Ida, Pingala and Sushmana. In Sanskrit these channels are called 'nadis'. Ida, Pingala and Sushmana are inside our Subtle Body, not the Physical Body. Ida carries the current of life force through the left side of the body, while Pingala carries it through the right. Sushmana carries the current in the middle of the spinal column. Ida rules the left nostril and Pingala rules the right. Ida is the calming, feminine, intuitive and cooling energy, while Pingala is active, fiery, male and heat-producing. Ida, Pingala and Sushmana meet together at six different places. Each meeting place forms a chakra. This is the melting pot for the trinity of creation. The Seventh Chakra, at the Crown, is our connection to universal consciousness; it is the gateway to liberation. This chakra is always open, if it was not our lives would not be sustainable. From the diagram below you can understand the route of these three energies and how they then go on to form the chakras.

Each chakra corresponds with a particular level of consciousness. In addition to this, every chakra has a close association with the endocrine (glandular) system within the body. Traditionally, chakras govern certain emotions, thoughts and desires. When in balance the chakras will reveal certain gifts that we, by birthright, should claim. When out of balance, we will begin to take on the shadow effects of the chakra, and if ignored we may become victim to sickness within that part of the body. Every word, thought and deed will reveal to you where your consciousness is residing within the chakra system. When you understand how it works, you will then be able to decide how to start working on areas of your life in which certain chakras seem stuck.

The chakra system has been divided into triangles. The lower triangle (First, Second and Third chakras) relate to our animal, instinctual selves, while the higher triangle (Fifth, Sixth and Seventh Chakras) to the more Divine aspects of ourselves. The Fourth Centre being the heart, is the mid-point of our human consciousness. It is this mid-point we need to aspire to if we are to move into the Aquarian Age at peace with ourselves. The Star of David, pictured below, is the perfect symbol of our quest in life. We need to raise the vibration of the lower triangle and pull down the inherent qualities of the Divine to reside at the heart, to be the full potential of a human being.

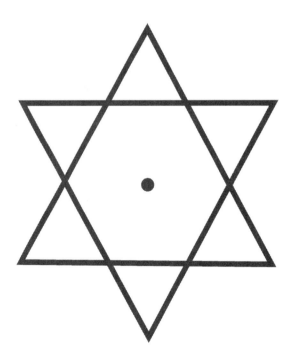

Muladhara

The First Chakra – foundations, elimination, security and habit.

This chakra is known as the Base, or Root, Chakra. It is located in the base of the spine. It is the most veiled to spirit, as it is deeply wrapped in the illusions of separateness, aloneness and tangibility. The First Chakra is our fundamental drive to survive. Its function in the body is elimination of our waste products. Not only is it our physical waste but also the removal of emotions and thoughts. It is the realm of our habits, fears and our instinctual behaviour that we use for survival. When the First Chakra is functioning well you will be steadfast, secure, trusting, stable, positively relentless and loyal. Thoughts that become obsessive, sadness that will not go, depression that is a lack of feeling all need the strength of the First Chakra to overcome. A strong First Chakra will incorporate the feelings of security, trust that all is well no matter what life throws up for us. A weak First Chakra can give way to deep psychological problems such as depression, grief and insecurity. Other signs of a weak First Chakra are being self-indulgent, greedy and egocentric. Holding on to the past for fear of the future is a sign of imbalance.

Location	Base of the spine
Function	Elimination, survival, grounding,
Element	Earth
Inner state	Stability
Glands	Adrenals
Body parts	Legs, anus, bones, large intestine
Malfunction	Obesity, haemorrhoids, constipation, sciatica
Colour	Red
Sense	Smell

Svadisthana

The Second Chakra – to feel, to desire, to create

Unlike the First Chakra, whose vision of the world is singular, secure and isolated, the Second Chakra requires others. Sexuality in the Second Chakra is not about self-stimulation, but the stimulation that occurs within oneself when with others. When the Second Chakra is well developed you will paint the world with passion, opinion and motivation. When the Second Chakra is weak the world seems flat; there is little passion and you lack opinion. Your body will feel limp and constricted. When the Second Chakra is overactive everything is sexual; there is sexual mania.

This chakra is located within the abdomen, midway between the pubis and navel. The major function of this chakra is procreation and creativity. In the body this chakra governs all the liquids: the circulation of the blood, the production of urine, menstrual flow and the production of seminal fluids. Blockages or imbalances in this area can cause disruption in any of these systems. Frustration, both sexual and creative, can be generated here when the life energies are blocked. When this chakra is balanced it brings a sense of self-confidence and creativity.

Location	The sacral plexus
Element	Water
Function	Pleasure, sexuality, procreation, creativity
Inner state	Self-confidence, well-being
Body parts	Womb, kidneys, reproductive system, circulation, bladder
Glands	Ovaries, testicles
Malfunction	Impotence, frigidity, uterine, bladder or kidney trouble
Colour	Orange
Sense	Taste

Manipura

The Third Chakra – the will of the Spiritual Warrior

The Third Chakra is the centre of energy, will power and control. It is associated with the region around the Navel Point. It is ruled by the element of fire. Of the three lower chakras this is the subtlest. It is the driving force to act and to complete the conceptualization.

A strong person at the Third Chakra will have a sense that their life and the quality of their life depend on what they do. There is deep confidence that they can shape, direct and develop what happens within their life. When this chakra dominates, that person will be exuberant and expressive. When the energy in the third is insufficient, a person has to compensate. You will be unable to finish tasks, you will be easily swayed by others and your sense of self-direction and self-determination will be underdeveloped. When the will is blocked we experience a tightening of the whole solar plexus area. The chakra will then not be able to release the energy, and so it will act as a dam, holding back feelings, needs and drives. There is inner turmoil, repressed anger and contained force. Eventually something snaps and there is an emotional scene. This chakra contains our raw emotions. Anger can remain trapped here for many years.

The Third Chakra is located behind the navel. In the body the Third Chakra governs the digestion, which transmutes food into energy.

Location	Behind the Navel Point
Element	Fire
Function	Will, power
Inner state	Intense emotion, laughter, joy, anger
Body parts	Digestive system, liver, spleen, stomach, small intestine
Malfunction	Ulcers, diabetes, eating disorders
Colour	Yellow
Sense	Sight

Anahata

The Fourth Chakra – love and awakening

The Heart Chakra is ruled by the element of air. It represents the opening of feelings, compassion and the capacity to love. It is the balance point between the flow of the upper energies of heaven and the lower flows of the Earth. The opening of the Heart Chakra will allow you to fully see others as important as yourself. The Heart Chakra is the centre of relationships and relatedness. The quality, degree and form of love assigned to the Fourth Chakra is quite different from personal love. It brings forth a particular quality of energy that pours from the Heart Centre. It is compassion that is universal and unconditional. The energy itself has the capacity to heal and change. Mother Theresa was, without doubt, a living embodiment of this force.

The Fourth Chakra resides in the middle of the breastbone. In the body it governs the immune system and the lungs. The ability to heal is associated with this chakra, along with the ability to touch. Your words and your smile will touch others. The path towards higher consciousness begins at this centre.

Location	Breastbone
Element	Air
Function	Love
Inner state	Compassion, love
Body parts	Lungs, heart, arms, hands
Glands	Thymus
Malfunction	Asthma, blood pressure, heart disease, lung disease,
Colour	Green
Sense	Touch

Vishuddha

The Fifth Chakra – speak and create

The Fifth Chakra is located in the throat. It deals with our verbal communication. The function of hearing is also attributed to this chakra. The Fifth Centre is associated with the thyroid and parathyroid glands. This chakra is entering into the miraculous and the mysterious. Ether is the element that rules this centre; the subtlest of all the elements. Ether is the condition of time and space to allow something to exist. The spoken word is the seed to manifestation. With the opening of this centre, you will know the very beginnings of cause and effect before you speak.

A strong Fifth Chakra will give you a strong and truthful voice. Your words will hold weight. You will not entertain mindless chatter. A weak Throat Chakra houses a weak voice, a quiet voice, and one who is afraid to speak up. Lying, dishonesty and fear of upsetting others by confrontation are symptoms of an imbalanced Fifth Chakra. Swallowing your words and keeping your truth down will lead to problems in the throat area.

Location	Throat
Element	Ether
Function	Creativity, communication
Inner state	Intuition, synthesis
Body parts	Neck, shoulders
Glands	Thyroid, parathyroid
Malfunction	Sore throat, swollen glands, colds, thyroid problems
Colour	Bright blue
Sense	Hearing

Ajna

The Sixth Chakra – to command

The Sixth Chakra is in the Brow Point. It corresponds to the pituitary gland. It is here, when you gain your intuition in terms of the direction, that you want to go. It is here that the major channels of energy meet (Ida, Pingala and Sushmana). This is the chakra associated with the Third Eye, the eye that gives you the depth and dimension within the subtle worlds. The Third Eye holds the knot of Shiva. To dissolve this knot is to attain a state of unity, to overcome duality; to realize fully that there is no separation between Self and everything else. As speech is to the Throat Centre, so visualization is to the Brow Chakra. This chakra has the power to manifest from thought alone. The awakening of this chakra brings such a state of consciousness that you will be able to communicate with your inner teacher, the source of wisdom within.

The pituitary gland is known as the 'master gland' and it governs twelve separate hormones within the body. It regulates sleep patterns, sexual maturation, repair of bodily tissue and breast-feeding.

Location	The brow
Element	None
Function	Direct perception
Inner state	Self-mastery
Body parts	Eyes, two hemispheres of the brain
Gland	Pituitary
Malfunction	Headaches, nightmares, defects of vision
Colour	Indigo
Sense	none

Sahasrara

The Seventh Chakra – the Universal Connection

The Crown Chakra is located over the top of the head, and it is associated with the pineal gland. The Seventh Chakra has key characteristics of humility, surrender and of 'bowing down' to the Infinite. The twin forces of Ida and Pingala have now been absorbed by the Sushmana at the Brow Centre; it is now the pure force of one at the Crown. The awakening of the Crown Chakra is at the heart of Buddhism, Sufism, Hinduism and yoga. It is the realm of enlightenment. Its association to the pineal gland is still a mystery. So far we know that this gland is connected to the amount of available light we receive. It is also connected to the amount of spiritual light that we receive. The Crown Chakra represents the potential for enlightenment that we all possess. The seven-fold pattern represented by the chakras system is the blueprint for spiritual development.

Location	Crown of the head
Element	None
Function	Union
Inner state	Bliss
Body parts	Cerebral cortex, brain, the whole body
Gland	Pineal
Malfunction	Alienation
Colour	Violet
Sense	None

The Eighth Chakra – the Aura

As you rise high above yourself, you imagine the radiant light of the aura surrounding your body like an egg or oval. This is often referred to as the shell that surrounds all the other chakras. It, too, is a chakra, a vortex of energy and a place to focus the flows of universal energy. When this field is strong you automatically filter out negative influences. When it is weak you seem vulnerable to everything that passes by or through you. A strong aura makes all the other chakras work better. The sensitivity that comes through the aura is connectedness; it interweaves you with the entire Universe. It establishes your sense of domain and fills the room with your presence. When the aura is strong and the chakras are aligned, your very presence will direct the forces in the Universe to fulfil your desires and needs.

The Three Knots

When you look at the symbolism of the chakras you will find that there are three knots that need to be penetrated for the path of kundalini to flow freely. Only consciousness can dissolve the three knots. Each of these three knots is represented by a Shiva Lingham, that which is surrounded by something symbolically in the chakras. The first one is the Knot of Brahman, which is in the First Chakra. The second is the Knot of Vishnu at the Heart Chakra. The third is the Knot of Shiva at the Brow Point. In each of these places all the three streams of energy come together and knot and entangle themselves into an energetic realm. As your awareness penetrates the first lower knot, you start releasing your attachment to all the sensations, the names and the forms of all things. You will begin to forge a new relationship to the senses and the sensations that come through them. Before you penetrate that knot every sense grabs your mind and seizes it, making it very difficult to be still and steady. All the meditations that stimulate the Navel Chakra will open up the fire that will eventually break through the first barrier to awakening.

As the second knot unties it adjusts the relationship to that which sustains. The meaning of Vishnu is 'the sustainer'. When it is still bound in a knot, you find yourself trying to establish your identity through relationships. This can either be personal relationships or a relationship to a tradition that binds you. As the knot is penetrated, you gain a lightness of heart and playfulness. You no longer feel attached to any of the forms in life. It will open up the ability to start hearing the subtle sounds or cosmic frequencies that yogis listen to in deep meditation.

Finally, there is the third knot at the brow. Here the knot is beyond the five elements. It is at this place that the Ida crosses over the Pingala nadis. When this opens, the breath balances in both nostrils equally for a time. It pierces you beyond the sense of time and the sense of lower identity. Yogi Bhajan always states that when you open this centre you will see the past, present and future. When this knot is still firmly tied, you may indeed gain powers, but you will be attached to them. So, this is a very challenging knot to overcome because many people believe they have opened it just because they are having psychic experiences. Their attachments to those realms betray them.

As the kundalini energy grows these knots are opened. These three gateways are one of the reasons that the three locks are so important. The Great Lock puts a slight pressure on all three knots, so that the Prana and Apana can balance in the Ida and Pingala channels. When this happens you will start to open the flow of energy into the depths of the knot, to eventually untangle the blockage. The Root Lock mixes the Prana and Apana and pulls the lower three chakras out of their slumber, by using the fire at the Third Chakra. The Diaphragm Lock works on the second knot at the heart. This works by pulling the fire at the Third Chakra up into the Heart Centre, which eventually pours into the Second Lock. When reciting mantra and after having applied both the diaphragm and Neck Locks, the *ojas* (cerebrospinal fluid) in the spinal column is concentrated and starts opening not only the Fifth Chakra but begins to penetrate the third gateway at the Sixth Chakra.

The Chakra Symbols

Illustrated below are the chakras:

First Chakra: This is associated with the qualities of stability and security. When it is functioning well the person will be comfortable and feel that all their needs are met. It is often pictured as a disc of red light.

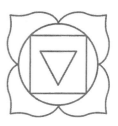

Second Chakra: This is the seat of creativity and sexual energy. It is usually pictured as orange. In balance the person can channel powerful reproductive energy to use for other creativity.

Third Chakra: This is the centre of power, energy and well-being. It is pictured as a golden yellow and associated with the Sun and fire. A strong navel bestows character, physical vitality and power.

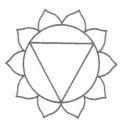

Fourth Chakra: This is the seat of compassion, love and free will. It is associated with green or sometimes rose pink. To live in the heart is to be true to Source. A strong Heart Chakra will also govern a strong immune system.

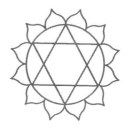

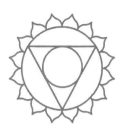

Fifth Chakra: This is where the poisons are purified, respiration is controlled and speech originates. It is perceived as sapphire blue. Its function ensures truthful speech, a pure and clean body and mind and some psychic facilities.

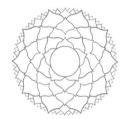

Sixth Chakra: This is the seat of intuitive awareness. This is the home of the true self. It is associated with indigo. You can insert your own spiritual guru within the symbol to provide you with guidance.

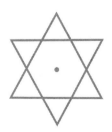

Seventh Chakra: This is often depicted as a 1,000-petalled lotus. This is your super-consciousness, your link with God and Universal consciousness. Its colour is violet.

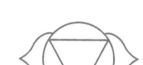

Eighth Chakra: This is the energy field of every human being. A strong aura ensures physical health and success. Wearing white expands the aura. We use the aura to project and protect ourselves.

How to Begin

This chapter will cover the actual application of Kundalini Yoga. There is an inherent depth to Kundalini Yoga, and there is also a tradition. To really attain the jewel embedded within the teachings, please follow the instructions carefully at all times.

Please consult a doctor and your teacher if you have any medical problems or are pregnant. When pregnant you can still practise yoga, *but* there are postures and breathing exercises that you should not do.

All medical conditions and any form of medication, prescribed or otherwise, *must* be made clear to your teacher.

It is always advisable to wear white cotton clothing, have a natural mat to sit on and to practise in a space that has enough room, good ventilation and is clean. Remember to switch the phone off, and to use a clock with a timer, so that you can do the precise timings necessary for all the postures and meditations.

Tuning In

Every Kundalini Yoga session always begins with chanting the Adi Mantra 'Ong Namo Guru Dev Namo'. By chanting this mantra in its correct form and consciousness, the student will open up to the Higher Self, the source of all guidance, and assess the protective link between the student and the consciousness of the Divine teacher.

The Adi Mantra

The Adi Mantra is always chanted at least three times, to open up the energy before the set begins. Even if you are only going to practise a meditation or mantra, it is still chanted. *Adi* means 'first' or 'primal'. It immediately centres you into the Higher Self, and calls upon this knowledge to guide you through the experience. It is an invitation to your Higher Self to take the helm and guide the course of the experience. Technically, it is the linking mantra to the Golden Chain. The Golden Chain is the inner spark of kundalini that is passed from person to person, teacher to student, guru to teacher, Cosmos and God to guru. Chanting this mantra will make you very receptive and sensitive to the messages of your body, mind and intuition. It immediately connects you to the long line of Spiritual Masters who have preceded us on the path.

How to Chant

Sit in Easy Pose, with your spine straight. Rub your palms together to stimulate the nerve endings in the palms. Bring your palms together into Prayer Pose. This is done by pressing both palms together, with the thumbs resting on your breastbone. Prayer Pose is one of the very best mudras for concentration, since within the palms are nerve endings that correspond to the left and right hemispheres of the brain. This brings an internal balance by regulating the logical hemisphere with the intuitive side. Press back with the thumbs just until you can feel your heartbeat. Slightly angle your palms upwards and outwards. Close your eyes and focus on the Brow Point (between the eyebrows). Take three deep breaths through the nostrils. This is to centre you and settle the mind. When you are ready inhale deeply and chant the words on the exhale. To begin with you may not be able to chant the entire mantra on one breath. You can therefore break the mantra after Namo, take a quick in-breath and continue chanting. Always chant the Adi Mantra at least three times.

Ong Namo Guru Dev Namo

The sound 'Ong' is created in the inner chambers of the upper palate and sinuses. The mouth is open to balance the resonance of the sound, but the actual sound comes out through the nose. Emphasize the 'ng' sound in the head and heart. The first part of Namo is short and rhymes with 'hum' and 'oh'. The 'oh' sound is held much longer. The first syllable of guru is pronounced as in the word 'good', while 'ru' rhymes with 'true'. The word Dev rhymes with 'save'.

When you have completed the tuning-in process, inhale deeply and hold the breath for a short time, and as you exhale feel all your worries and tensions being carried away with the breath.

The Adi Mantra translates as 'I call on the Divine wisdom'.

To really understand the correct way of chanting, *see page* 231 for information on where to buy tapes, CDs and further books on kundalini and other related subjects.

Mental Focus

To fully appreciate and receive the benefits of each posture and meditation you will need mental focus. Unless you are directed to do otherwise, always focus at your Brow Point. With your eyes closed, mentally locate the area between your eyebrows and concentrate there. The eyes will gently roll upwards and inwards to correctly rest at this place. Remain aware of your breath, your body posture, your movements and any mantra that you may be using. Every time your eyes or concentration move off this point, just continue to bring it back.

Linking Breath with Mantra

To gain a deeper experience of Kundalini Yoga you can mentally recite a mantra with the breath while practising the exercises. This is a very powerful technique that engages the mind, while the Higher Self gets on with the healing that needs to be done within the individual.

A mantra is a sequence of sounds designed to direct the mind by their rhythmic repetition. To fully utilize the power of mantra, link the mantra with your breath cycle. A common mantra is 'Sat Nam'. This mantra means 'truth is my identity'. Mentally repeat 'Sat' as you inhale, and 'Nam' as you exhale. In this way you will filter your thoughts so that each thought has a positive resolution. Mantra is also a great way of keeping up with the more physical exercises and adds depth to the performance of the simpler ones.

Pacing Yourself

Kundalini Yoga exercises involve rhythmic movement between two or more postures. With experience you will be able to speed up and rapidly move from one posture to another. Always follow the breath with the movement. Begin slowly, keeping a steady rhythm. Increase gradually, being careful not to strain. Usually the more you practise an exercise, the faster you can go. Just be sure that your spine has become warm and flexible before attempting the rapid movements. It is important to be aware of your body and to be responsible for its well-being. If you should get dizzy, reduce your speed to a more moderate pace, until you feel you are able to speed up again.

Concluding an Exercise

Unless otherwise stated, an exercise is concluded by inhaling and holding the breath briefly, then exhaling and relaxing the posture. While the breath is being held, apply the Root Lock, contracting the muscles around the anus, the sex organs, and the Navel Point. This consolidates the effects of the exercise and circulates the energy to your higher centres. Do not hold the breath to the point of dizziness. If you start to feel dizzy or faint, immediately exhale and relax. Remember to keep your spine straight, and your face, neck and shoulders relaxed when applying the Root Lock.

Relaxation

An important part of any exercise is the relaxation following it. You can take between one and three minutes to completely observe the effects within the body and mind. Be sure to follow the instruction of the kriya as occasionally there will be a sequence of exercises when there is no rest and you will be instructed to flow from one posture to another. To relax after an exercise you should adopt either Easy Pose or lie on your back or stomach, depending on which position is most convenient for you and which requires least movement to get into. When resting you should completely let go of your body; there should be a feeling of surrender with no tension anywhere. Check that your shoulders are relaxed and that you are not clenching your teeth together. I always suggest that you part your lips and let your jaw go loose. Also check your forehead and eyebrows for any tension, and just let your face drop. Continue breathing long and deep through your nostrils, and just allow your body to balance. Try imagining that you are a pond, and someone has just thrown a pebble into the middle (your Navel Point). Imagine the ripples of water freely travelling up to your chest and head and down through your legs and feet. Just observe the mind and do not get involved with any thoughts.

At the end of the kriya, before the meditation, there will be a period of deep relaxation. This is always done in Corpse Pose, with a blanket or shawl over you. When in deep relaxation your blood pressure slows right down and your temperature may fall slightly. Rather than becoming attached to the thought that you are getting cold, cover yourself up. The duration of the deep relaxation is standardized at 11 minutes. Again the idea is to let go of your body and your thoughts. Keep your breath at a natural pace and just allow your body and mind to process the energy that you have built throughout the kriya. Sometimes you may even fall asleep. This is great. Don't fight it; just allow the body to do what it needs to. You may find that the body jumps and twitches. Again this is perfectly normal as it is the nerve endings adjusting and balancing.

Grounding

When time is up, slowly inhale and exhale a couple of times to bring yourself back into your body. Then begin to move your fingers and toes, and then slowly start to rotate your wrists and ankles in one direction and then the other. Bring your feet together, point your toes and then inhale and stretch your arms overhead. With your arms outstretched inhale and bend your right knee to your chest, and exhale the knee over to the left side. You can help your right knee down with your left hand. But keep your right arm outstretched and on the floor. Come back to centre and repeat on the other side. Bend both knees and begin to rub the soles of your feet and palms together. Next bring your knees to your chest and rock from side to side on your spine. Then bring your nose up to your knees, with a rounded spine start to roll up and down the spine. Be sure that your spine is rounded and that you are rocking smoothly along the length of the spine. Just do this for half a minute. Then do one big rock and come into Easy Pose.

If you are going to do a meditation, do it now, after the deep relaxation and before the closing sequence.

Closing Sequence

Sit in Easy Pose with a straight spine and with the Neck Lock applied. Again rub your palms together. Then bring them together into Prayer Pose at your chest. This is a very important part, as it is again confirmation to yourself that 'Truth is my identity'. It is also the final section of the grounding sequence.

Inhale and exhale three times. Inhale to chant 'Sat Nam'. The word 'Sat' needs to be seven times longer than the 'Nam'. The way you can do this is to visualize the beginnings of the word

'Sat' in the First Chakra. As you continue to chant, see the 'Sat' interweaving up through all the chakras until you come to the top of the head. Imagine the sound current following the path of kundalini as it penetrates every chakra, and that way you can guarantee that it has passed through all seven centres. The 'Nam' is short and can be visualized moving down from the Crown into the Heart. It is traditional for this mantra to be repeated three times. But you can do this as many times as you like.

When you have done this, place your palms on the floor and bring your forehead as close as you can to the ground. Spend a few moments in prayer, and give thanks to the wonderful experience that you have just been given. Again, it is very important to bow your head, as this will ensure that the blood floods back into the brain and leave you feeling completely grounded and centred.

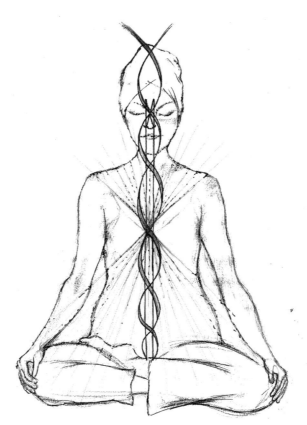

Important things to remember

- Never extend the times given, though you may decrease the times. These sets have been specifically designed to have a certain effect on the body and mind. Bear in mind that we are playing with the power of the atom, and this has to be respected. Yogi Bhajan has given us a safe and easy technique. To go beyond his guidelines is entering unknown territory.
- Never change the kriya or the sequence of the movements. If there is a posture that you do not like, do not miss it out. Just do all that you can, even if it is just for a few seconds. Again, the kriyas form a sequence that raises the energy and then guides it to certain points in the body and mind. By missing one out you will be not be following the direct tried-and-tested method.
- Women, please note that during the heaviest days of your period avoid doing any inverted postures, any breath that involves pumping the navel, any heavy abdominal exercises and only do a very light Breath of Fire, making sure that you do not pump the navel.

Basic Sitting Postures

The correct name for a posture or pose in yoga is *Asana*. Asanas are designed to stimulate the glands, organs and body awareness. Asanas often apply pressure on the nerves and acupressure points, which reflex back to the brain and body for certain effects. Initially these basic postures may be difficult to maintain, but practise as often as possible. Whenever you can, perform the posture just for a couple of minutes.

The most common sitting asanas are:

Easy Pose (Sukasana)

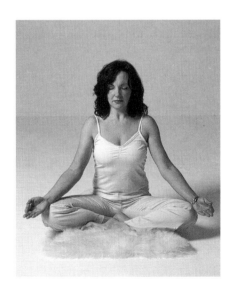

Sitting on the floor, place one heel at the perineum, with the sole against your inner thigh. Then bring the sole of the other foot to rest against the shin of your opposite leg. It is very important that your feet connect with your thigh and shin. Concentrate on relaxing your knees to the ground. Eventually, with practice, your hips will loosen and your knees will go to the floor. It is often a good idea, if this pose is uncomfortable, to sit on a cushion or on yoga blocks. This will raise your bottom, allowing your spine to straighten and your knees to be lower than your hips.

Always ensure that your spine is straight and that there is a sense of elevation within your whole body.

Variation: You can try the normal cross-legged position that we all did at school. Place your feet under opposite knees. Pull your spine up straight.

Lotus

Sitting on the floor, lift your left foot on to your right thigh, then place the right foot on the left thigh, as close to the body as possible. The right leg is always on top. Straighten your spine and lift your chest. Press the lower spine slightly forwards. This position will make you feel 'locked in place'. Once you are in it you can meditate very deeply and the position will maintain itself. There are very few kriyas that use this posture, but it is still recognized that it is the very best position for deep meditation.

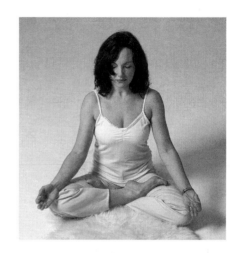

Half Lotus

Sit in Easy Pose and pull your top foot all the way across on to the upper thigh instead of leaving it near the ankle. Pull your spine straight

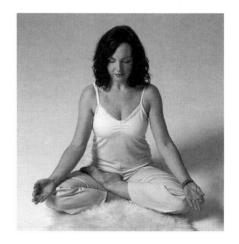

Rock Pose (Vajrasana)

This asana is well known for its benefits for the digestive system. It also makes you as solid and balanced as a 'rock'.

Start by kneeling on your knees, with the top of your feet on the ground. Sit back on your heels. The heels will press two nerves that run into the lower centre of each buttock. Keep your spine pulled straight. If this is uncomfortable for you, place a cushion between your bottom and your feet.

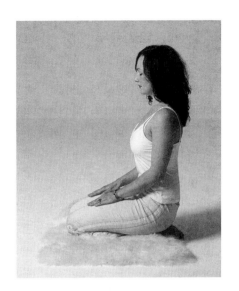

Celibate Pose (Hero Pose)

With your feet a hip-width apart, kneel and sit between your heels. This posture channels sexual energy to be used throughout the whole body and pull your spine straight.

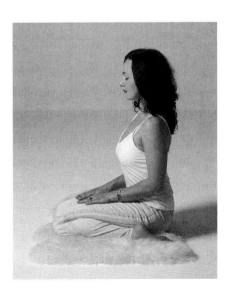

Sitting in a Chair

If these sitting postures are not possible due to a back injury or some other difficulty, you can still practise yoga by sitting in a chair. Make sure that it is a chair with a firm back support, as you will still need to have your spine straight. You will also have to make sure that both feet are flat on the floor and the same distance apart as your hips.

Corpse Pose

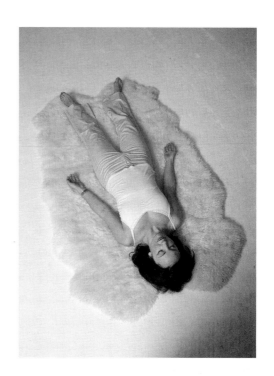

For this position you will need to lie down on your back. Make sure that your legs are slightly apart, with your ankles flopped open to the sides. Your arms are at your sides, palms face up. Your shoulders are dropped and there should be no tension in your body. Your teeth are not touching and your lips are slightly parted. Move around until you feel that even weight is balanced on both sides of your body. Make sure your body is in a straight line.

This position totally balances the body and mind; it is well worth getting into this position when you first get into bed. If you can sleep like this you will be balancing your entire body and mind.

Warm-Ups

Before beginning any kriya in Kundalini Yoga there is always a short time for warm-ups: usually 20 minutes. These exercises are vital for preparation of the spine for yoga, to open the lungs and to settle the mind. All these warm-ups work up the chakra system, opening and stimulating the energy centres, from the base of your spine to your head. Warm-ups are still performed with the eyes closed, breath coming through the nostrils and still maintaining a focus with the eyes held at the Brow Point. Again, after each exercise observe the effects by keeping the focus at the Brow Centre, and observing the feelings/thoughts within the body and mind. After 20–30 seconds move on to the next posture.

Spinal Flex

Sit in Easy Pose with a straight spine. Place your hands on your outside leg, near the shin. Inhale and flex your spine forwards, making sure your chin is still parallel to the ground. Your chin should jut forwards and your bottom is pushed out. As you exhale push your spine back until it is rounded. Your chin should be parallel to the ground. Continue this flexing of the spine for one minute.

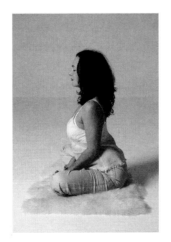
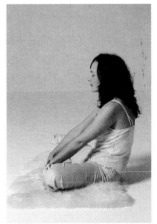

Butterfly

Sitting on the ground bring the soles of your feet together. Interlock your fingers and hold on to your toes, bringing your feet as close to the perineum as possible. With a straight spine start to flap your knees up and down about 10–15 cm (4–6 in). Keep the breath long and deep. (One minute.)

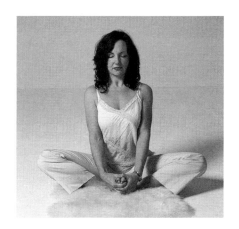

Hip Raises

Lie on the ground with your knees bent and open the same width as your hips. Place your feet squarely on the floor, again the same width apart as your hips. Holding on to your ankles, or with your palms face down on the floor, inhale and raise your hips up. Hold for a couple of seconds, then exhale as you lower them again. Continue lifting your hips up and down. (One minute.) To end, inhale up and hold for 15 seconds and exhale down.

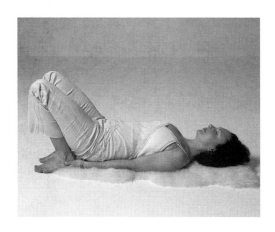
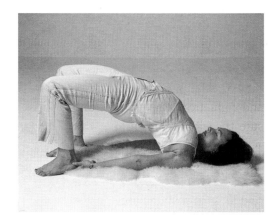

Stretch Pose

Still lying on your back, bring your feet together and point your toes. Raise your legs 15 cm (6 in) and raise your arms just above the hips, palms facing each other. Make sure that your back is pressed into the floor at all times, to avoid lower back injury. If your back rises up, you can pull your knees up until it goes back to the floor. Lift your head up and look at your feet. Do Breath of Fire, thrusting the navel on each exhale. (One minute.)

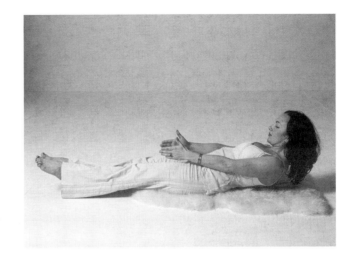

Spinal Twist

Sitting in Easy Pose with a straight spine. Place your thumbs at the back of the shoulders with the fingers at the front. As you inhale twist left and as you exhale twist right. Continue twisting left and right from the hips making sure the elbows are in line with your shoulders. (One minute.) To finish, inhale to return to centre, hold the breath a couple of seconds, and exhale your arms down.

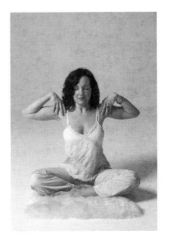
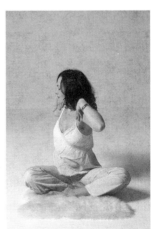

Shoulder Shrugs

In Rock Pose, inhale your shoulders up to your ears, and exhale back down. Your palms rest on your thighs, arms relaxed. Continue inhaling up and exhaling down. (One minute.) To finish, inhale up and hold and then exhale down.

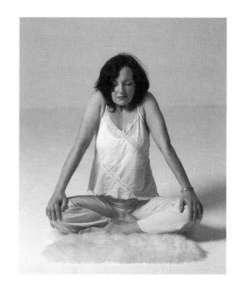

Neck Rolls

Still in Rock Pose, start to gently rotate the head with a long deep breath. Take care as you bring your head back. The main stretch is as you bring your ear-lobes to your shoulders and your chin down on to your chest. After one minute, change direction for a further minute. To finish, inhale, centre and exhale.

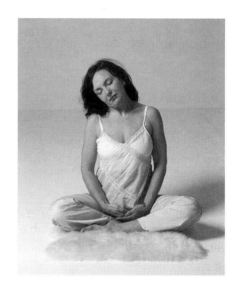

Cow-Cat

On all-fours, with your knees directly under your hips and your hands under your shoulders, inhale, allowing your spine to drop downwards, raising your chin as high as you can into Cow. As you exhale, lift and round your spine, bringing your chin to the chest into Cat. Continue inhaling up and exhaling rounded. (One minute.) To finish, inhale up into Cow and hold for 15 seconds. As you exhale bring your forehead down to the ground and stretch forwards with your arms still on the ground.

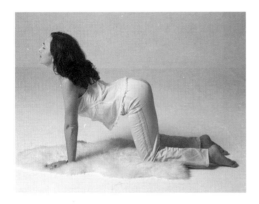
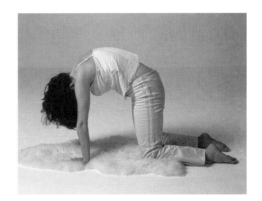

Life Nerve Stretch

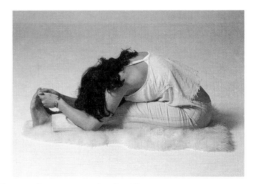

With both legs stretched out and together, inhale and stretch your arms up, then bend at the hips to grab your toes. If you can reach, pinch the big toe with your thumb and forefinger. Holding on to your toes, shins, or wherever you can reach to, inhale and straighten your spine and exhale down as far as you can go. Make sure your legs are straight and the backs of your knees touch the floor. (One minute.) To finish, inhale up and exhale down, stay down, with the breath held out, for a couple of seconds.

Alternate Life Nerve Stretch

Open your legs as wide as you can, with the backs of your knees touching the floor. Inhale up and exhale down and reach for your left foot. Again, if you can, pinch the big toe. Holding on to the left leg, continue inhaling up and exhaling down. (One minute.) Then change to the right. (One minute.)

To finish the life nerve stretches, hold on to both feet, inhale up, and exhale the forehead down to the ground. Continue for one minute. To finish, inhale up and exhale down and bring your forehead to the ground, hold the breath out for a couple of seconds. Then slowly come up.

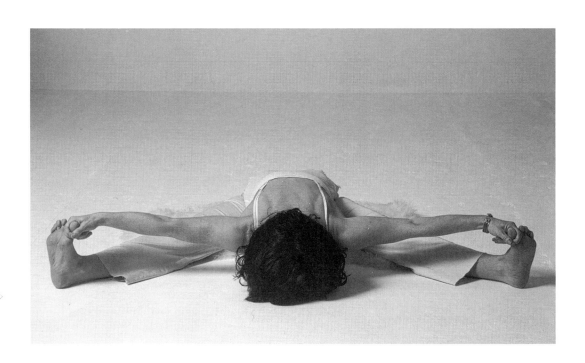

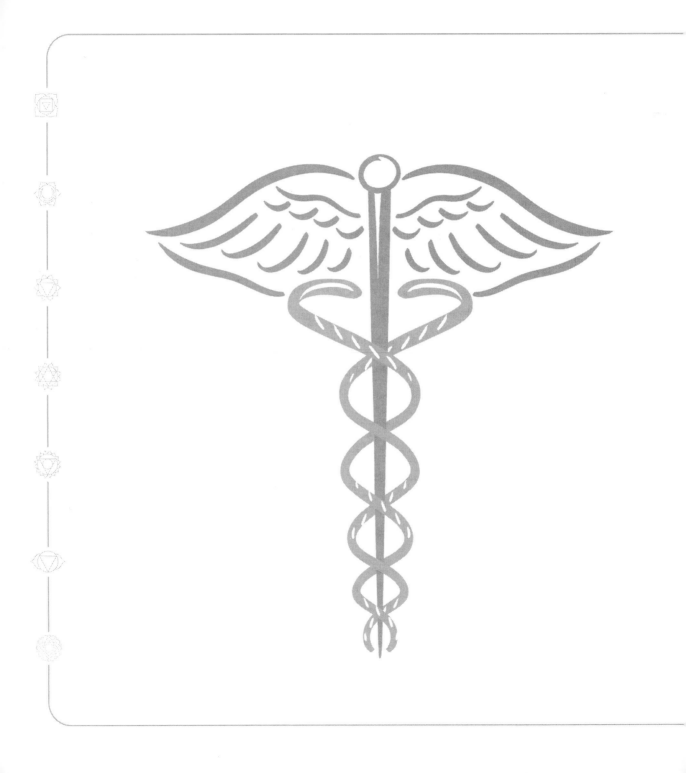

part three

The Practice of
Kundalini Yoga

The Body Sets

The Body

These kriyas are designed to work within the physical systems of the body. Each posture is an exercise, a meditation and a diagnostic instrument. As an exercise, the posture is used to isolate specific muscles, to pressurize specific points that act as reflex triggers to enhance the functions of the glands and organs, and to redirect, flush or increase circulation.

As a meditation, the posture creates a special link and foundation between the body and the mind. Each posture stimulates an area of the body as the meditation technique employed begins to release emotional masking and blocks. The frequency of the mind's thoughts and the emotional tone of the experience are intimately tied to the posture that you use.

As a diagnostic, particular postures may give you signals of pleasure or of discomfort and pain that indicate conditions of the muscles, glands or emotions.

There are two forms of pain common to the practice of yoga postures. The first is the normal distress that comes from fatigue or effort when extending a muscle or stimulating a nerve. This pain is recognized when extending an arm out parallel to the ground for a certain amount of time. The arm becomes heavy and sore and you feel that you cannot hold it out any longer. This pain is not harmful and will dissolve with concentration, a slow controlled breath and a welcome flood of endorphins. These types of pain reflex are often a signal about the condition and balance of the glandular and nerve systems.

The second type of pain comes from structural problems, bruises, inner organ difficulties and referred pain due to a variety of injuries and illnesses. It will not just pass, nor should it be ignored or 'worked through'. Stop the posture and check with your medical adviser. Examples of this are disk problems, infections, swollen glands or sprained ligaments. In less severe cases, a simple adjustment of the posture or a substitute posture is helpful.

When practising Kundalini Yoga within the group, remember that the whole group's auras merge into one. So even if you miss certain postures but maintain the breath, mantra and focus you will still benefit from the group energy of the posture. Imagine you are doing the exercise perfectly well. The mind will accept this and the benefits of the posture will still have the required effect.

Bear in mind that yoga is union, not battle.

For best results, find a set that resonates with you and practise the same set every day for 40 days, with no breaks. If you do break, start again at day one. The time period of 40 days has always had mystical significance. It is known to be a natural period for humankind to break a habit or pattern within the psyche. It takes another 40 days to plant a new pattern, and a further 40 days to seal it. The reason it works is because you will have worked through all eight chakras with the five elements. Eight chakras multiplied by five elements equals 40 days. To practise a set or meditation for 120 days will wipe a pattern from your psyche and set up a new behaviour that is reflective of the true Self.

The times are shown to provide you with a goal. To begin with attempt to do every exercise for at least one minute's duration. With practice, slowly work up to the designated times. Remember that if you halve the time limit on one posture, you must remember to do the same with all the other postures in the set. Never go beyond the designated time given.

Removing Body Blocks

This is a very powerful set that will get to work on any blocks in the body that manifest as disease or pain. We all know of our personal weaknesses within our bodies, be it our digestion or lungs, but we do not have to live with them as our inherent birth defect. The weakness is there for a reason, to show us what we have to work on in this lifetime. As the weakness is dissolved all the mental and emotional issues linked to the particular area will also come up into your awareness to be released. For further understanding on disease within the body study the chapter on Chakras (see page 82), to see the connection between the mind, body and emotions.

SIRI DATTA

1. Easy Pose: Sit in Easy Pose and raise your arms over your head with your palms facing. Move your raised arms in a clockwise circle. This movement opens up your shoulders. Allow the breath to develop its own pace for the exercise. Move fast. (Four and a half minutes.)

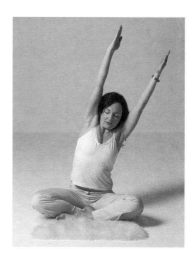

2. Easy Pose: Stretch your arms straight up, with the palms facing ahead and bend at the waist, touching your hands and forehead to the ground. Rise back up and continue for two and a half minutes.

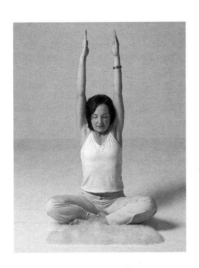 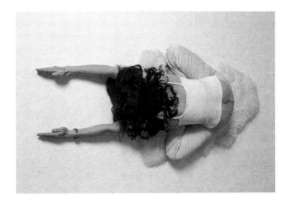

3. Stand up and put your hands on the ground. Jump up and down in this 'all-fours' position. Concentrate on your navel, pulling up on it to power your jumps. (Two minutes.)

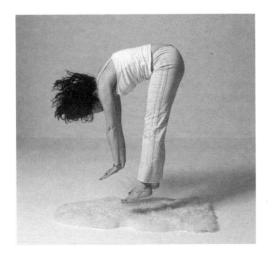

4. From the standing position, exhale as you bend forwards and touch the ground. Rise up with the inhale and bend backwards. Continue this sequence, making sure that the head does not drop backwards but remains upright as you lean back. Keep your arms straight and open the same width as your shoulders. Palms should be facing forwards. (One minute.)

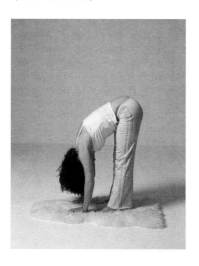 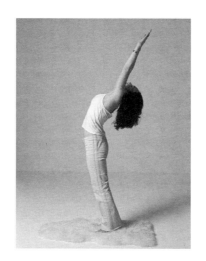

5. With your hands on your hips, alternately criss-cross your legs. Move quickly and continuously. (Two minutes.) Your eyes should be closed, but they may be opened to maintain balance. If so keep them focused on a point on the floor.

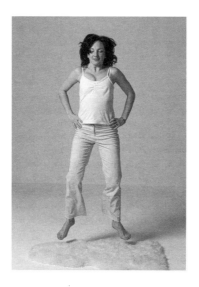

6. With your arms overhead and the palms facing each other, criss-cross your arms and legs. Keep your arms straight. (Two minutes.)

7. Easy Pose: Make fists of your hands and hold them level at the Heart Centre, making sure the fists do not touch. Bend your elbows so that your forearms are parallel to the ground. Hunch up your shoulders, pull up on your rib cage and alternately roll each shoulder forwards. Keep your spine straight and upright. (One minute.)

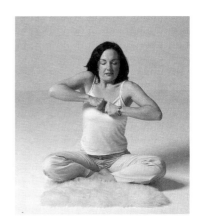

8. Stretch Pose: Lying on your back, bring your legs and feet together. Raise your legs 15 cm (6 in) and point your toes. Raise your arms so that they are parallel to the ground and turn your palms to face each other. Raise your head and shoulders up while looking at your toes. Begin Breath of Fire for one and a half minutes.

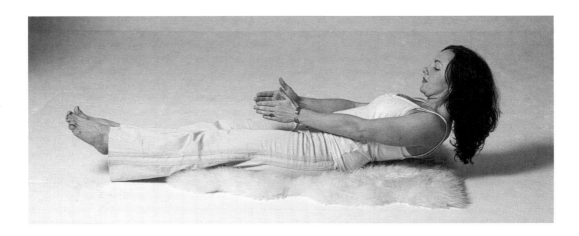

9. Lock your knees to your chest and roll back and forth on your spine. Make sure your feet do not cross. (30 seconds.)

10. Roll back and forth on your spine in either Easy Pose or Lotus. (One and a half minutes.)

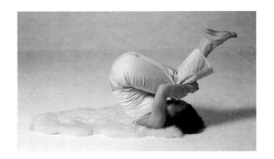

11. Come into the all-fours position again, as in Exercise 3. Dance to Sat Nam, Wahe Guru, Indian version. (Two minutes.) This is a dance to stretch out the body.
Move the hips, arch your feet, and press down with your hands. Stretch the arms, ribcage and lower back. Turn your head left and right. Move everything.

12. Lie down flat and pull your knees alternately to your chest. Pull your left leg to the chest on the inhale and pull your right leg to your chest on the exhale. Keep your outstretched legs parallel to the floor. Continue this movement for one and a half minutes. The Navel Point is balanced with this stretch.

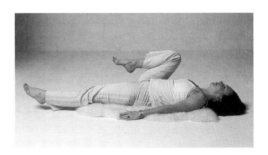

13. Still lying on your back, bring your arms up as if to clap, but make no sound. Open your arms wide and repeat it. The kriya exercises the chest muscles. Powerful breath. (One minute.)

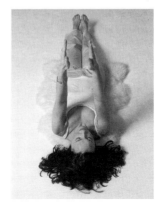

14. Corpse Pose: Lie flat on your back with your arms by your sides and relax totally. Concentrate on your Sixth Chakra and project out from the Brow Point. (Nine minutes.)

15. Stay in this position and sing along with Sat Nam, Wahe Guru, Indian version. (Two minutes.)

16. Roll your wrists and ankles, rub your hands and feet, and roll on your spine. Wake your Self up. You could do the grounding exercises.

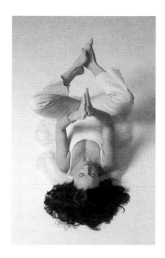

17. Stand in Tree Pose. Bring your left foot to rest against the inside of your right thigh. Keep your hips straight and brings your arms overhead into Prayer Pose. Keep your eyes focused on a point on the floor. Long, deep breathing. (45 seconds.) Change legs and repeat Tree Pose for 15 seconds.

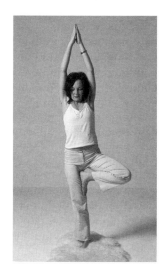

18. Use both hands to massage your face, scalp and ears deeply and vigorously. (One and a half minutes.) Massage your chest, shoulders, and armpits. (30 seconds.) Flex your spine. (30 seconds.) Stretch your arms. (10 seconds.)

19. Relax deeply.

Boosting Your Immune System

This set works on boosting the immune system. Working alongside is the lymphatic system, which is responsible for the white blood cells, known as antibodies, which fight all forms of infection and pollution within the body. Rich sources of these antibodies are produced in the armpits and under the jaw. When you are ill these areas become tender as the body boosts the production of these vital cells.

When both internal systems are working well and are being flushed regularly you can fight off anything.

It is advisable to practise this set at the beginning of any illness.

SIRI DATTA

1. Easy Pose: Bend your elbows and tuck them into the sides of your ribs. Make sure that your forearms and hands point straight up, with all your fingers touching and your palms facing each other. Push one arm strongly up and out to a 60-degree angle, while the other arm remains in the starting position. Keep the remaining arm rigid and steel-like. Then return the outstretched arm and raise the other arm up and out. Continue this intentional and focused movement. Work hard to do this exercise. Breath is long and deep through the nostrils. Continue for 10 minutes.

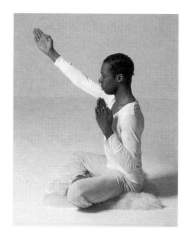

2. Easy Pose: Extend both arms up and out at a 60-degree angle with the palms facing. Keep your arms straight as you criss-cross them in front of your face. Move quickly with Breath of Fire. (One and a half minutes.)

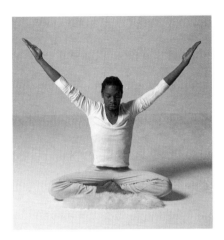 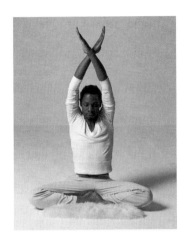

3. Easy Pose: Extend both arms out in front of you, parallel to the ground, with the palms facing up and cupped. Keep the arms together at all times. Visualize a pool of water as you dip your hands in the water and then splash it up and over your head. Continue with this movement. Breathe powerfully through your mouth. (Two and a half minutes.)

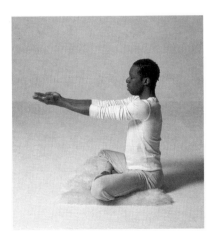 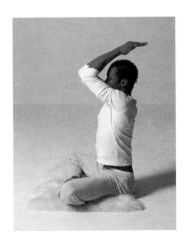

4. Lie down on your back, with your arms at your sides, palms face down and lift both legs up and over your head into Plough Pose. Return your legs to the floor and continue leg lifts into the Plough Pose. Breathe long and deep through the nose. (Two minutes.)

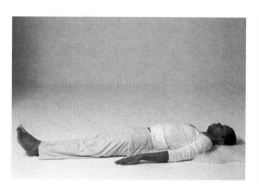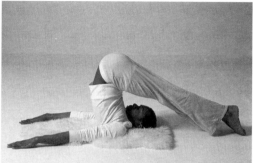

5. Lie down on your back and interlock your fingers under your neck. Spread your heels 15 cm (1 ft) apart. Begin to lift your body up on to your heels and shoulders and then drop your body back down. Continue this jumping movement from the hips, as vigorously as you can. Do not bend the knees, but move from your thighs and ribcage. Continue for three and a half minutes.

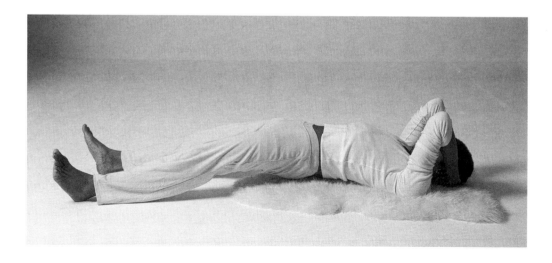

6. Still on your back, lift your legs up and grab your toes, keeping your legs straight. If you cannot reach your toes, hold at the backs of your calves or the backs of your thighs, ensuring that your legs remain straight. The whole of your torso, neck and shoulders are relaxed and on the floor. Open your mouth and breathe through your throat. (One minute.)

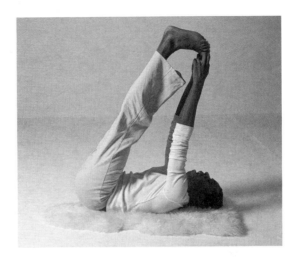

7. Baby Pose: Rest your forehead on the ground, with the full weight of your head supported and allow your spine to relax over your thighs. Keep your buttocks on your heels. Make sure that your arms are behind you with the palms face upwards. Go to sleep listening to 'Naad' by Sangeet Kaur. After 11 minutes come up into Easy Pose and place your right palm over your left, held at the Heart Centre, and sing along with the music for five minutes.

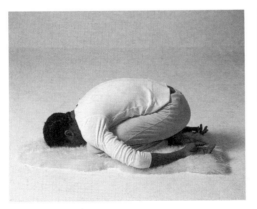

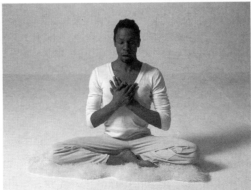

Unleashing Your Navel Power

This kriya takes you directly to the source of your personal power, which lies within the Navel Point. This storehouse of strength, when utilized, will give you the will power, endurance and stamina of a warrior. When you feel stuck, practise this set and everything will begin to work out for you again.

SIRI DATTA

1. Lie down on your back and lift both legs up to 30 degrees. With you face down at your sides, begin to move and shake your legs. Keep your legs straight, but shake and vibrate your ankle and knee joints. Breathe long and deep through your nostrils. Begin to chant along with the mantra 'Har Har Har Gobinde' by Nirinjan Kaur and Guru Prem Singh. (Four and a half minutes.)

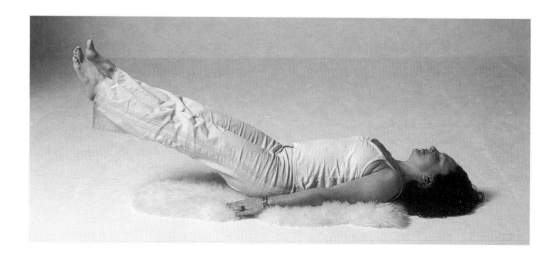

2. Celibate Pose: Make sure your buttocks are on the floor. Extend your arms, with your hands slightly cupped, making sure all the fingers touch, including the thumb pad connecting up with the first finger. Begin to extend your right arm as you pull back the left. Make sure your eyes remain closed. This movement is very powerful and intentional. Allow your body to move from the waist with the arm movement. Continue to chant along with the same mantra as for Exercise 1. (Two minutes.)

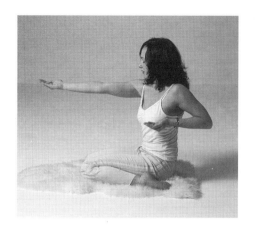

3. Celibate Pose: Raise your arms above your head, with your palms facing forwards, and then bring them down to the floor to hit the palms on the ground either side of your knees. Continue rising up with straight arms and then striking the ground. Hit the ground with all your body weight. Move to the rhythm of 'Har Singh, Nar Singh, Neel Narayan' by Nirinjan Kaur. (One minute.)

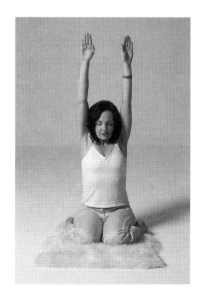 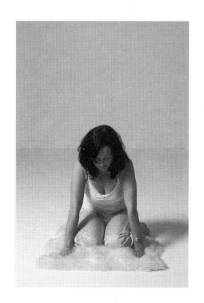

Then raise your arms overhead, interlocking your fingers with your index fingers extended. Sit quietly and meditate on the mantra. Keep your arms straight and pull up from the spine. After one minute begin to chant the mantra loudly from the Navel Point. Continue for another three minutes.

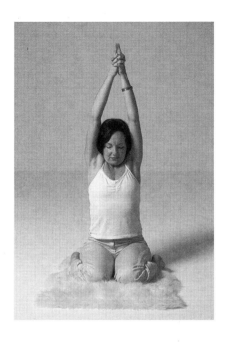

4. Celibate Pose: Lie back on the floor, with your legs still in Celibate Pose. Continue to hold your hands in the same mudra, but place them on the Navel Point with the first fingers pointing straight up. Continue to chant for three minutes.

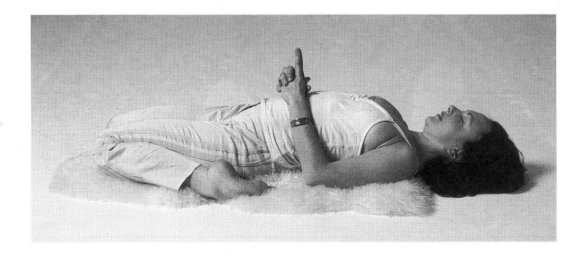

5. Rock Pose: Bring your palms together into Prayer Pose at the Heart Centre. Do this exercise with Ragi Sat Nam Singh's 'Jaap Sahib'. Initially hold your hands at the heart for the introduction prayer. Sing from your Heart Centre. When the Ragi sings the lines that begin with 'Namastang' or 'Namo', bow your head down to the floor with your hands either side of your knees. Stop at 'Chachri Chand'. (Three and three-quarter minutes.)

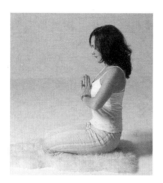 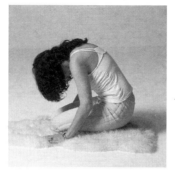 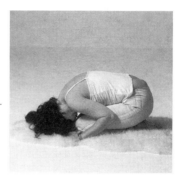

6. Hans (Swan) Kriya: Sit on your heels in Rock Pose, with your hands on the floor either side of your knees. Push back with your arms to round off your spine, bring your chin to your chest and extend the back of your neck as you bring your head down to the floor. Lower your total upper body weight on to the tops of your thighs as your head bows down. From this position arch your spine and neck up as in Cobra Pose *(see page 108)*, rising up into the sitting position and begin rounding your spine outwards again. Continue this movement of arching, rounding and stretching the spine for 108 repetitions. Make sure to stretch your entire neck and spine.

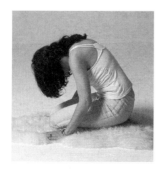 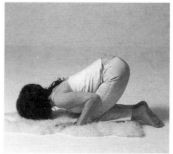 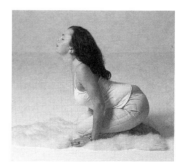

Detoxification

This set will get your energy moving again. When energy becomes stagnant a blockage will build up and if allowed to accumulate, will eventually manifest into the physical body as disease or pain.

This kriya will leave you feeling energized, light, spacious and re-vitalized. This is an excellent set to practise when embarking on a cleansing diet or lifestyle change. It is not just the physical by-products that will be cleared out, but the mental and emotional toxins that are just as important to get rid of.

SIRI DATTA

1. Lie down on your back, with your legs straight and your heels together. Keep your heels together as you spread your feet apart. The right foot points to the right and the left foot points to the left. Then close your feet so that they once again face upwards. Continue quickly, opening and closing your feet, keeping your heels together. The palms are face down. (Four minutes.)

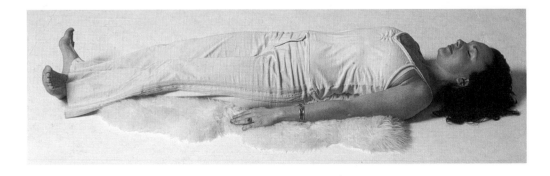

2. Remain on your back, interlock your fingers under your head, raise your legs up about 60 cm (2 ft) and scissor the legs up and down, without letting the heels touch the floor. Keep your legs straight and do not bend your knees. This exercise dissipates inner anger when you do it vigorously. (Four minutes.)

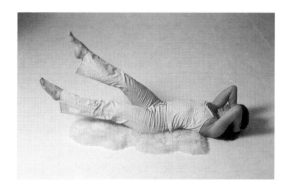

3. Lie down on your stomach, with your palms under your shoulders and stick your tongue out as far as it will go. Exhale through your mouth and push your upper body into Cobra Pose. Your hips need to remain on the floor and the goal is for your elbows to become straight. However, it is all right to bend your elbows to ensure that your hips remain on the floor and to keep your back strong. As you push up, open up your throat as you pull your head back. Inhale through your mouth as you lower yourself back down to the floor. Continue keeping your breath and movement strong. This exercise removes toxins from the body. (Six and a half minutes.)

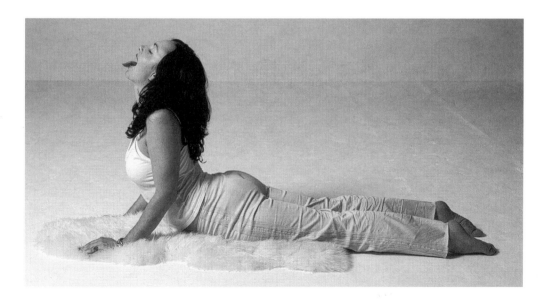

4. Turn over on to your back and bring your knees to your chest. Inhale as your knees touch your chest and raise your arms 90 degrees (parallel to each other). Then exhale, straighten your legs and lower your arms as you bring your feet to the floor. Continue this movement vigorously. (Three minutes.) This is a controlled movement and you should avoid making a noise when your arms and legs touch the floor.

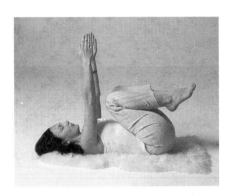 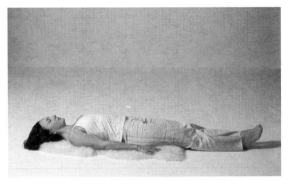

5. Easy Pose: Sit in Easy Pose with your hands on your knees and revolve your torso around the base of the spine. This churning movement is done in a counter-clockwise direction. Keep your spine straight as you rotate on your hips. Move as quickly as you can during the last minute. (Three minutes.)

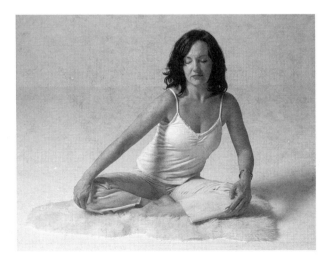

6. Stand up. Bend over and grab your ankles. While holding on to your ankles, squat down, with your buttocks resting on your heels. Inhale as you come up and straighten your legs. Exhale as you squat down. Continue this movement for two minutes.

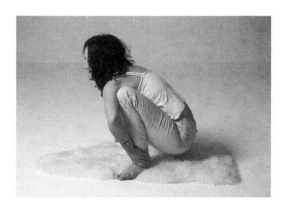 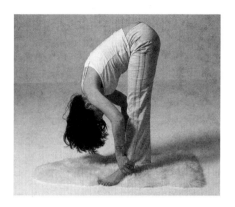

7. Easy Pose: Sit comfortably in Easy Pose, with your spine straight. Chant 'Sat Nam, Sat Nam, Sat Nam, Sat Nam, Sat Nam, Sat Nam, Wahe Guru'. One repetition of the mantra takes 7–8 seconds. Continue chanting for 11 minutes. To finish, inhale deeply and stretch your arms overhead with your palms touching in Prayer Mudra. Hold your breath 20–40 seconds as you stretch your spine upwards. Exhale. Repeat this sequence two more times.

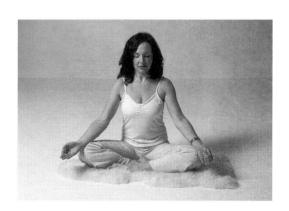 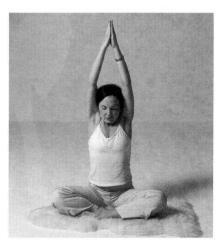

For Unknown Cause of Sickness

This is a very heavy set that will get to work on whatever is causing you dis-ease. Allow yourself enough time for deep relaxation afterwards. This is a very powerful kriya that works thoroughly on deep-rooted imbalances within the body and mind. Be prepared for anything afterwards!

SIRI DATTA

1. Cow Pose: Come on to all-fours and raise your left leg as high as you can. At the same time, raise your right arm straight up. This posture will balance the body and strengthen the Apanic energy. (Three minutes.) Inhale and raise the opposite arm and leg. (Two and a half minutes.)

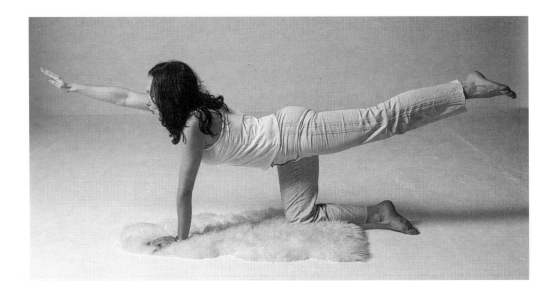

2. Sobagni Kriya: Come on to your knees and put your arms up straight over your head. Bend backwards from the navel and move your arms and neck in a circle; your shoulders will move but your knees will not. This is called Sobagni Kriya, the kriya of virtue. (Two minutes.)

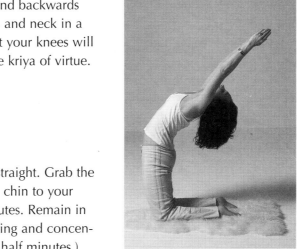

3. Sit down and stretch your legs out straight. Grab the bottoms of your feet and bring your chin to your knees. Hold for two and a half minutes. Remain in this position with long, deep breathing and concentrate on your Third Eye. (Two and a half minutes.)

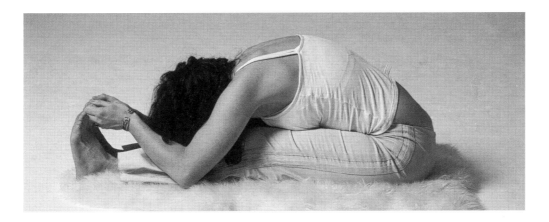

4. Corpse Pose: Lie on your back and deeply relax every part of your body while you project your energy out of your Third Eye. Be aware of letting go of your body, surrendering to releasing the sickness and pain. Visualize the dis-ease leaving your body. (Six minutes.)

The Mind

When our insecurities and fear attack together, the normal outcome is depression.

YOGI BHAJAN

Every human being belongs to Infinity and creativity. Kundalini Yoga balances out the glandular system, strengthens the nervous system, and enables a person to harness the energy of their mind and emotions. It is a technology that allows a person to bring equilibrium to their being, control to their physical structure and to experience their infinite Self.

The following sets are working within the arena of the mind. Clearing the sub-conscious, releasing outdated patterns and addictions, letting go of false ideas about ourselves, quieting the chaos and dissolving the restraints we have placed upon ourselves. It is the mind that traps us, stops us in our tracks with its false fears and illusions of the Self. It is here that intentional work needs to be done, to see through the false beliefs and boundaries.

The time limits are there to act as a goal. You can either attempt to practise each posture within the set for a minute, or you could halve the times on all the postures in the set. Never attempt to go beyond the time limits.

When working on the mind, it is always a good idea to keep a journal to document the changes within your belief system. The journal can record how the many changes will begin to take place. You may begin to notice less stress, positive decision-making, you will begin to throw off your insecurities and start to develop a healthy acceptance of yourself.

As you work within the arena of the mind, you will start to become aware of a state known as 'mindlessness'. This is when the mind stream stops briefly and the illusion is dropped. For a brief moment we become aware of our true essence, and deep inner peace is resonated throughout the whole body and psyche.

Mental Balance

Regularly practising Exercises 1 and 2 for three minutes each, and doing 108 frogs (Exercise 3) can achieve a clean bill of health mentally and physically.

HARIJOT KAUR KHALSA

1. Bow Pose: Lying on your stomach, reach back and grab your ankles and arch your body up like a bow. If you cannot reach your ankles, you could always use a towel to catch your feet. Keep lifting the chest and opening the throat throughout. After two minutes stick out your tongue as far as possible and breathe heavily through your mouth (this is called the Breath of the Lion). Continue for one and a half minutes.

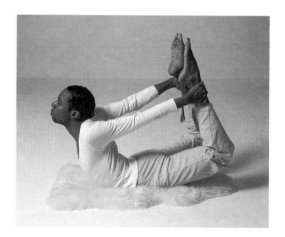

2. Camel Pose: From a sitting position on your heels, reach back and grab your ankles. As a variation you can either reach for your heels, or in the very beginning stages place your hands on the lower back to support the body as you bend backwards. Arch your body upwards and drop your head as far backwards as you can. Once again, stick out your tongue and begin Breath of the Lion. (Two minutes.)

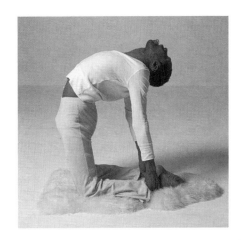

Both Exercises 1 and 2 stretch the thigh muscle. Pain in this area during these exercises indicates that the calcium–magnesium balance is out and that mental balance is also impaired.

3. Frog Pose: Squat down, with your buttocks on your heels. Your heels are off the ground but touching each other. Your fingertips are on the ground between your knees and your head is up. Inhale and straighten the legs, raising your buttocks high while keeping your heels off the ground. The head goes towards the knees. Exhale and return to the squatting position. Continue for a total of 108 repetitions. To begin practice you could aim for 26 repetitions, and then on to 52, with the goal being 108. Relax for five minutes.

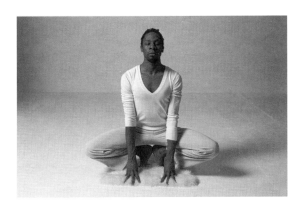
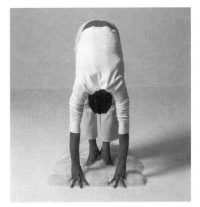

4. Celibate Pose: From a sitting position on your heels move your heels out to the sides so that your buttocks are resting on the floor. You can use a yoga block or cushion to sit on initially. Spread your knees as far apart as possible. Interlock your hands behind your back. From this position lower your torso towards the floor and rise back up, moving your shoulders from side to side, weaving like a snake. As you move forwards raise your arms up behind you as far as they will go. Continue this movement for three minutes.

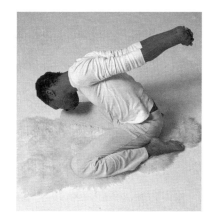

5. Lie on your back and bring your knees to your chest and lock your arms around your knees. While holding yourself in this posture bounce your body up and down on the floor. Just do all that you can. Keep your body moving. (Seven minutes.) Ancient yogis practised this posture to eliminate sexual imbalance.

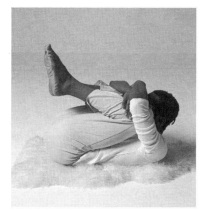

6. Easy Pose: Sit like a yogi in Easy Pose, with your spine straight and your hands resting on your knees. Inhale and powerfully exhale the breath so that the sound of the breath leaving the nostrils sounds like 'Har'. Pump your navel so that the exhalation goes from the navel to the nostrils. Your rib cage will lift with the power of the breath. (Three to five minutes.)

7. Relax deeply on your back. (Ten minutes.)

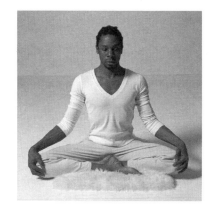

Relieving Inner Anger

Inner anger is destructive and dangerous to ourselves and to others. It will prevent you from having functional relationships, success in your life and eventually will manifest as dis-ease within your body.

Stored anger poisons the mind and body, the resentment and bitterness causes venom to build in the body and this venom will eventually start to eat you up – literally. Your inner anger will attract others into your life with the same problem and together you will fight and destroy each other.

This kriya will open up an outlet to allow the anger to pass through and out of your psyche. Intend for this to happen, and it will.

SIRI DATTA

1. Corpse Pose: Lie down flat on your back in a relaxed posture, with your arms at your sides, palms up and legs slightly apart. Pretend to snore. (One and a half minutes.)

2. Still lying on your back, keeping your legs out straight, raise both legs up to 15 cm (6 in) and hold with long, deep breathing. This exercise balances anger. It pressurizes the navel to balance the whole system. (Two minutes.)

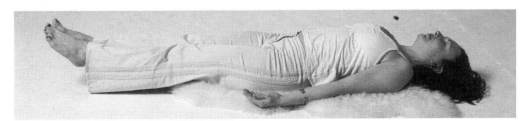

3. Remaining in this posture with your legs raised 15 cm (6 in), stick out your tongue and do Breath of Fire through your mouth. (One and a half minutes.)

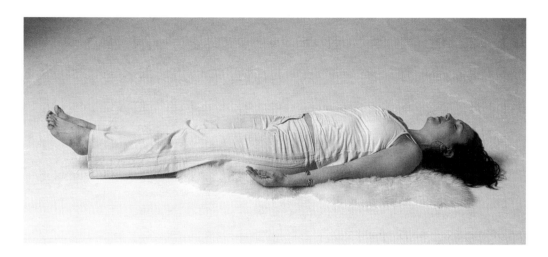

4. Still lying on your back, lift your legs up to 90 degrees, with your arms on the ground by your sides, palms facing down. Keeping your legs straight and raised, begin to hit the ground with your palms, using all the anger you can tap in to. Beat hard and fast. Allow it all out now! Two and a half minutes.

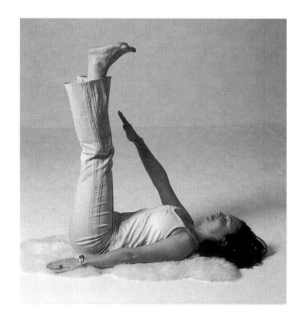

5. Still on your back, bring your knees to your chest, and stick your tongue out. Inhale through your open month and exhale through your nose. (Two minutes.)

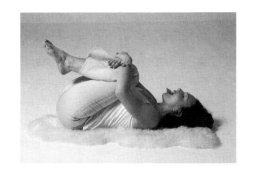

6. Celibate Pose: Sit in Celibate Pose, buttocks on the floor between your heels. Cross your arms over your chest and press them hard against your ribcage. Bend forwards and touch your forehead to the floor as if you were bowing. For two and a half minutes move at a pace of approximately 30 bows per minute. For the last 30 seconds speed up and move as fast as you can.

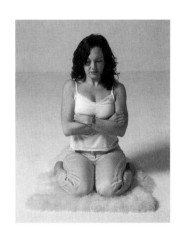

7. Sitting with your legs together, straight out in front of you, begin to beat all parts of your body with open palms. Legs, arms, chest, lower back, neck – everything. Move fast. (Two minutes.)

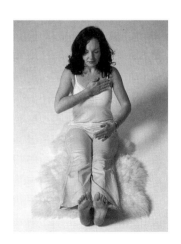

8. Stand up. Bend forwards, keeping your back parallel to the ground, let your arms and hands hang loose. Remain in this posture and sing for three minutes. 'Guru Guru Wahe Guru Guru Ram Das Guru' was played when Yogi Bhajan taught this class.

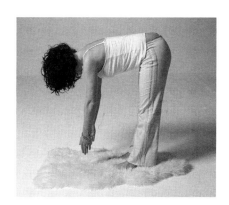

9. Cobra Pose: Continue singing and come into Cobra Pose, keeping your elbows straight, hips on the floor and continuously stretching your spine. (One minute.) Then begin circling your neck while still in Cobra Pose, still continuing to sing. (30 seconds). Maintaining Cobra Pose and still singing, begin kicking the ground with alternate feet.

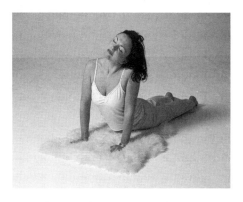 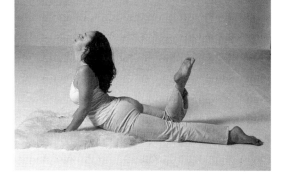

Continue for another 30 seconds.

10. Easy Pose: Sit in Easy Pose and close your eyes. Stretch your arms over your head, keeping your elbows straight; interlock your fingers with your index fingers pointing straight up. Begin Sat Kriya. (One minute and 15 seconds.)

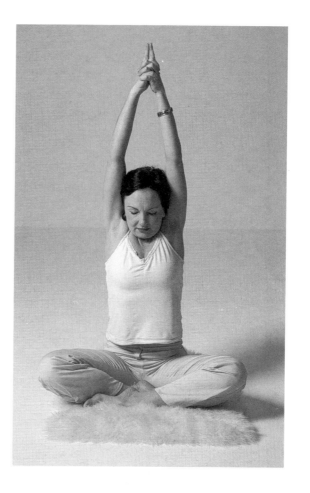

11. Corpse Pose: Lie down in Corpse Pose and sleep for five minutes.

Overcoming Tiredness

These exercises are for when you feel tired, sluggish and heavy. If you wake up feeling tired then this will be the kriya for you. Practise this kriya every morning until you begin to feel the benefits. If this is an overwhelming problem, check your stress levels and diet.

SIRI DATTA

1. Lie on your back with your legs together, palms face down. Begin to move your feet alternately forwards and back at the ankle, pointing and flexing the feet. (30 seconds.)

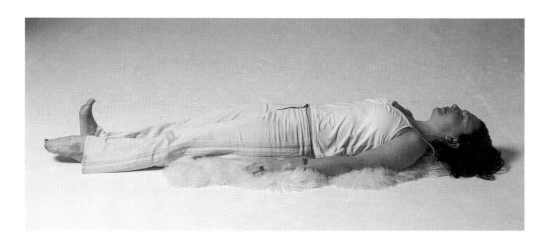

2. Sill on your back, raise and lower your knees alternately. (30 seconds.) Sometimes the circulation in the lower body becomes sluggish while you are asleep.

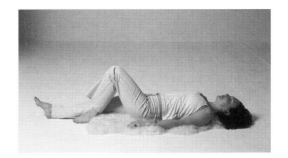

3. Still lying on your back, move your shoulders from side to side. Bring your shoulder up towards your ear as you pull the opposite shoulder down towards the feet. Continue raising alternate shoulders for one minute.

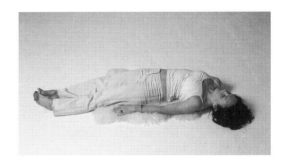

4. Clasp your knees to your chest with your arms. Lift your head and rotate your neck. Make sure you bring your chin to your chest. (30 seconds.)

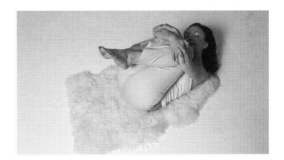

5. Stretch Pose: Lie down on your back and bring your feet together. Lift your legs 15 cm (6 in) and point your toes. Hold your arms at your sides slightly above the hips, palms facing. Raise your head and stare at your feet. Hold this position until the Navel Point begins to tremble and you feel you cannot stay up any longer. Relax. Repeat this exercise twice more. You can do this exercise for a total of three times or for three minutes, whichever is shorter.

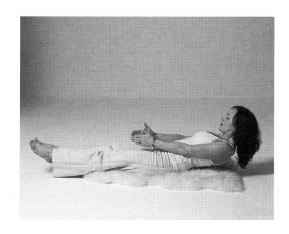

6. Cat Stretch: Lie on your back with your arms stretched out, inhale and bend your left knee. Exhale as you bring your left knee to your right side, still keeping your arms on the floor. Stay in this position with your spine fully open and breathe deeply. Come back to centre and stretch the other side. (30 seconds.)

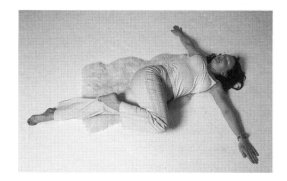

7. Sit up with your legs stretched out straight. Grab your toes. Raise and lower your torso, bringing your head to your knees. Keep your spine straight; do not bow your head. Inhale up and exhale down. (30 seconds).

8. Relax.

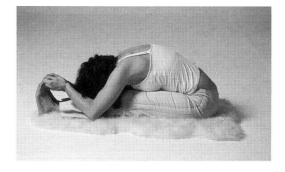

Beyond Stress

Stress is everywhere in the modern world, we cannot get rid of it, yet we can counterbalance its negative and dangerous effects. Chronic fatigue and attempts to self-medicate using various stimulants are signs that stress has led to poor adrenal function. This kriya is very beneficial in strengthening the adrenal glands and releasing long-term effects of stress from our body. It also improves digestion, balances the nervous system and brain hemispheres, helps alleviate fear and invigorates the body.

YOGI BHAJAN

1. Camel Pose: Open your knees the same distance as your hips, with the tops of your feet on the floor, lean back and grab your heels. If you cannot reach your heels, support your hips with your hands and lean backwards. Open up the front of your body, especially the chest and throat. Keep pushing forwards with the hips and pelvis. Allow your head to drop backwards. Breathe powerfully. Inhale deeply to fill the lungs and as you exhale pull the navel back towards the spine. Make sure to breathe one complete breath every two to three seconds. Continue for four minutes.

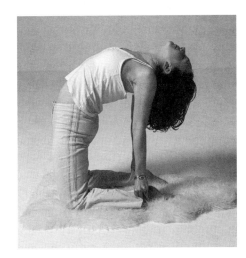

2. Crow Pose: Open your legs slightly wider than your hips, angle your feet slightly outwards and squat down. Your feet need to remain flat on the floor and your spine needs to remain straight. Work towards having your feet parallel and facing forwards. Extend the arms out in front and make fists with your hands. Maintain tension in the arms and fists. Begin to move your arms up and down quickly, one arm rising up 30 degrees as the other descends 30 degrees. Continue for two minutes.

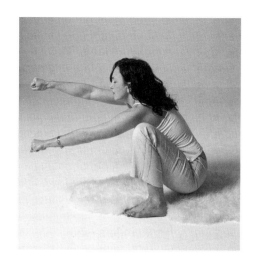

3. Lie on your back, interlocking your fingers behind your neck at the hairline. Open the elbows towards the floor. Raise your legs, hips, buttocks and torso off the floor, and then allow your body to drop down hard on to the floor. Continue for four minutes.

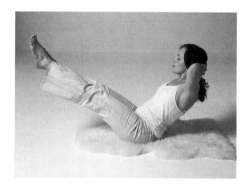

4. Easy Pose: Extend your arms out to the sides with your palms facing down. Keep your arms straight and move in a straight line like a see-saw motion. Every time your right arm lowers towards the floor, slap the ground four times. At the same time raise your left arm and also making the slapping motion to the chant 'Har Har Har Hari'. Chant powerfully from the navel for three minutes.

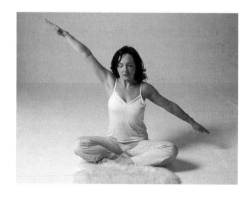

5. Easy Pose: Continue to move your arms as in Exercise 4, with the mantra 'Har Har Wahe Guru'. On the fifth beat, on the word 'guru', do a quick double-strike with your hands. Continue for three minutes.

6. Repeat Exercise 5, chanting the 'Har Har Wahe Guru' mantra twice per side for three minutes each time.

7. Continue to chant 'Har Har Wahe Guru' as you proceed through the following postures. Do each posture for 30 seconds.

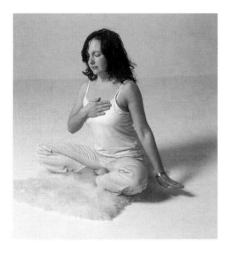 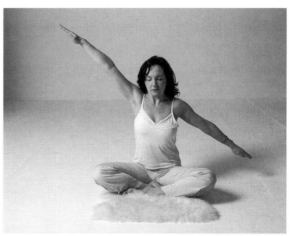

   a)   Place your right hand on your heart and tap the ground with your left hand.
   b)   Continue with both arms, as in Exercise 4.
   c)   Continue the same as in Exercise 7A
   d)   Continue the same as Exercise 7B
   e)   Continue the same as Exercise 7A

This exercise is a great workout for the brain, as it strengthens the electromagnetic field. The upper arm movement is good for maintaining youthfulness and the motion of the lower arm brings you increased energy.

8. Easy Pose: Extend your arms straight in front of you, parallel to the ground with your hands in fists. Powerfully move both arms alternately 30 degrees above and 30 degrees below parallel. Move fast and strong, like a machine. Begin with Breath of Fire, then substitute with the mantra 'Sa-a Ta-a Na-a Ma-a' in rhythm with the movement. Continue for two minutes.

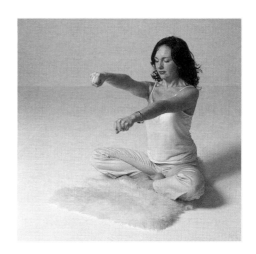

9. Easy Pose: Bring your hands in Gyan Mudra to rest on your knees. Breathe long and gently, experiencing peace and compassion. Meditate and feel healed deep within. Begin to sing 'Dhan Dhan Ram Das Guru' or any other KY Mantra or 3HO music *(see page 231)*. Sing from the heart and continue for five to ten minutes.

10. Corpse Pose: Rest deeply for 10 minutes.

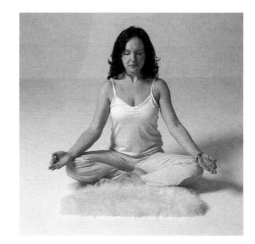

The Soul

These kriyas are often more subtle, leading you to experience the Self. As you will encounter, the times are longer and there are fewer exercises in one set. You will be working on the higher frequencies of your Self, fine-tuning your sensitivities to allow the Soul to shine through. Try to lose yourself in the exercise; let go and surrender. Allow the magic of the set to heal you, in ways you could not have imagined.

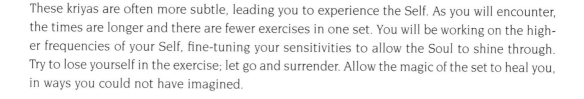

Open to Love

This exercise will strengthen the nervous system and open the heart.

YOGI BHAJAN

If we all did this kriya there would no more war, hatred, anger or fear. When a human being is taught this exercise only love will live in the heart, all else ceases to be…

SIRI DATTA

The blood becomes purified as it is flushed throughout the whole body. 15 minutes of this exercise will keep you young, happy, beautiful (inside and out) and healthy.

1. Corpse Pose: Very slowly and very graciously lift up your left palm and kiss it gently in the centre and then return your arm to the floor. Continue this same slow, loving movement with your right arm. When you kiss, really feel the tenderness and the blessing. Continue for 11 minutes.

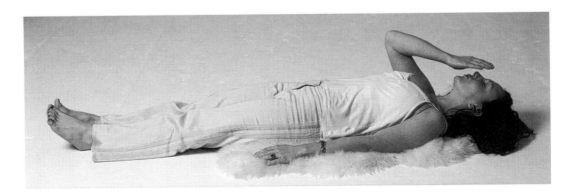

2. Bring your knees to your chest and place your hands in the fold behind your knees. Raise your legs up and over as if you were coming into Plough Pose. Keep your hands steady as you return your knees to your chest. Continue raising your legs over the body and back to the chest for a further 5–15 minutes.

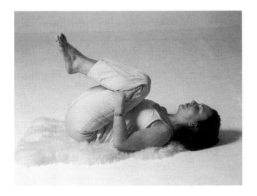 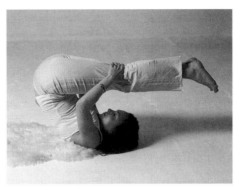

Relax completely.

Becoming Like Angels

This kriya is for those who experience the 'longing' to make a difference for the evolution of humankind and the planet. It is for those whose heart cries when they see humankind destroy itself along with all other innocent life. It is for those beautiful souls who have incarnated here from the Angelic Realm with a job to do, but are too confused with all the glories of human life to know where to begin. This kriya will put you in tune with your Angelic Essence, where you will be able to access your mission and your message.

SIRI DATTA

1. Easy Pose: Stretch your right arm for-
    wards with the palm facing down. Pat
    the air, moving up 30 degrees and
    returning parallel to the ground. Move
    from the shoulder and pat at a speed of
    thirty times per minute. Create a steady
    rhythm. Keep your left elbow bent, with
    your left upper arm near the ribs. The
    palm faces forwards and the fingers
    point straight up. Close your eyes.
    Inhale through your nose and exhale
    through your mouth. Breathe slowly,
    heavily and deeply. (Six minutes.)

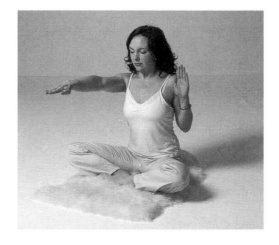

    People who have regularly done this exercise have become angels in their own right.
    This exercise will cause some pain as it realigns the patterns of the body. You are
    hurting yourself so that ill health does not hurt you.

2. Change hands and repeat the exercise. (Three minutes.)

3. Relax and roll your shoulders. Loosen up. (Two minutes.)

4. Easy Pose: Bend both elbows, keeping the upper arms close to the ribs. Keep your wrists bent and the palms facing upwards. The hands point away from the body diagonally. Your eyes focus on the tip of your nose. Inhale through the nose and exhale through the mouth as fast and as powerfully as you can. Hold your body in perfect balance. There will be tremendous pressure on the chest. (Five and a half minutes.) This exercise can get rid of chronic illnesses that you may have developed over the years.

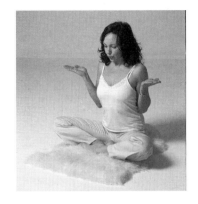

5. Easy Pose: Rhythmically hit the ground in front of you with both your hands at the same time. Chant 'Har', using the tip of your tongue. Use the power of the Navel Point to chant and time the chant in rhythm with the clapping of the ground. (Six and a half minutes.) To finish, inhale, hold the breath 15–20 seconds, tense all your muscles and press your hands against the ground with the entire weight of the body. Exhale explosively through the mouth. Repeat this sequence two more times.

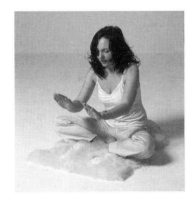

6. Take two minutes to recover from the powerful effects of this kriya. Do not meditate or be silent. Stretch, walk around and talk before resuming normal activities.

Creating Self-Love

Exercise 1 is called Reverse Adi Shakti Kriya. Here you are mentally and hypnotically blessing yourself. This self-blessing affects and corrects the magnetic field. If you are storing any issues preventing you from experiencing self love, then this kriya will show you this in no uncertain terms. You may experience this as pain in your arms and upper back, you may feel incredibly emotional or there may be an outburst of frustration or anger. Stay with it, and realize that you are letting go of false judgments about yourself.

SIRI DATTA

NB: There are no breaks between exercises.

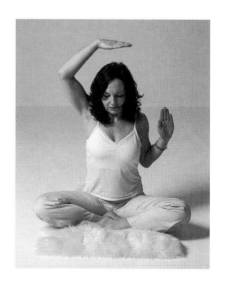

1. Easy Pose: With a straight spine, hold your right palm 15–22 cm (6–9 in) above the top of your head. Your right palm faces down, blessing you. Your left elbow is bent, with the upper arm near the rib cage. Your forearm and hand point upwards. The left palm faces forwards, blessing the world. Your eyes are closed and focused at the Lunar Centre, in the middle of the chin. Breathe long, slowly and deeply with a sense of self-affection. Try to breathe one breath per minute. Inhale 20 seconds, hold 20 seconds, and exhale 20 seconds. (Eleven minutes.)

2. Easy Pose: Extend your arms straight out in front, parallel to the ground, palms facing down. Stretch out to your maximum. The eyes are closed and focused at the Lunar Centre, in the middle of the chin. The breath is long, slow and deep. (Three minutes)

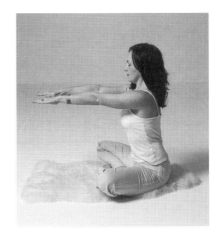

3. Easy Pose: Stretch your arms straight up, with the palms facing forwards. Do not bend your elbows. Your eyes are closed and focused at the Lunar Centre. The breath is long, slow and deep. (Three minutes.) To finish, inhale and hold your breath for 10 seconds, while you stretch your arms upwards. Stretch from your buttocks. Tighten all the muscles in the body. Exhale. Repeat this sequence two more times.

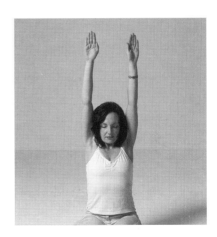

Self-Renewal

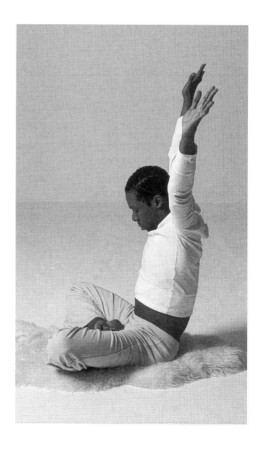

When you cannot live with yourself a moment longer – practise this set.

SIRI DATTA

1. This exercise balances the sugar and
   sodium in your body.
   Easy Pose: Lean the spine backwards,
   allowing your head to be slightly back,
   with your chin tucked in and your chest
   pushed out. Extend your arms up and out
   to a 60-degree angle. Spread your fingers
   with the palms facing forwards. Be relaxed
   in this posture, but hold it still. You may
   experience pressure in the shoulderblade
   area. Begin Breath of Fire from your Navel
   Point. After three minutes, open your
   mouth and stick out your tongue as far as
   you can, as you continue Breath of Fire for
   another two minutes.

2. This exercise stretches the spine and keeps you youthful and healthy.

   Easy Pose: Stretch your arms overhead with your palms in Prayer Pose. Keep stretching your spine and armpits. Pull your spine and ribcage upwards. Fight gravity with your own will power. Under no circumstance let your palms separate. If you need to rest, lower your arms, but keep your palms together. Continue holding this posture for three to five minutes.

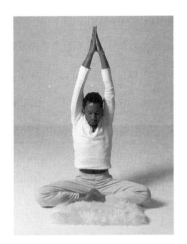

3. This exercise balances the glandular system.

   Easy Pose: Bring your thumbs to the mound below your ring (third) finger and then close all your other fingers over the thumb to make fists. Lean back as in Exercise 1. Stretch your arms out to the sides and begin to move your arms quickly in small backward circles. Continue to make small backward circles as you raise up your arms and lower them again. There should be pressure between the shoulderblades. Continue this movement for seven minutes.

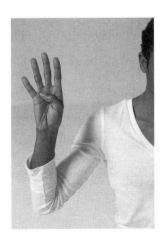
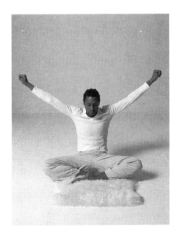
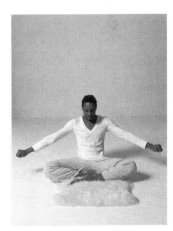

4. This exercise loosens up your spine and balances the left and right hemispheres of the brain.

   Easy Pose: Stretch your arms out to the sides, forming a straight line. Turn your left palm down, while the right palm faces up. Keeping your arms in a straight line begin to raise one arm up as you lower the other. Continue this see-saw movement as quickly as you can for three minutes.

5. Easy Pose: Bend your elbows so that your hands are by your ears. Place the thumb on the mound underneath your little finger, keeping your other fingers pointing straight up. Your fingers should not be touching each other. Close your eyes and look at your chin and begin to watch on your internal screen one of your fantasies or dramas. Relax and meditate for 11 minutes. Breathe long, slow and deep. After 11 minutes, inhale, hold your breath and tighten every muscle of your body as you remain in the posture. Exhale and repeat this two more times.

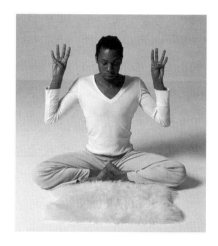

6. Get up and dance! Shake, jump, vibrate and gyrate every part of your body to flush the energy of the previous meditation through your whole body. (Three to five minutes.)

7. Easy Pose: Bring your hands into Prayer Pose and place your thumbs gently in the eye sockets where they join the bridge of the nose. Do not press too hard. Chant 'Ong Namo Guru Dev Namo' with Nirinjin Kaur's tape for three minutes. Afterwards inhale, hold the breath for 10 seconds and exhale. Repeat this two more times.

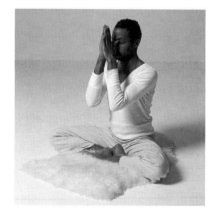

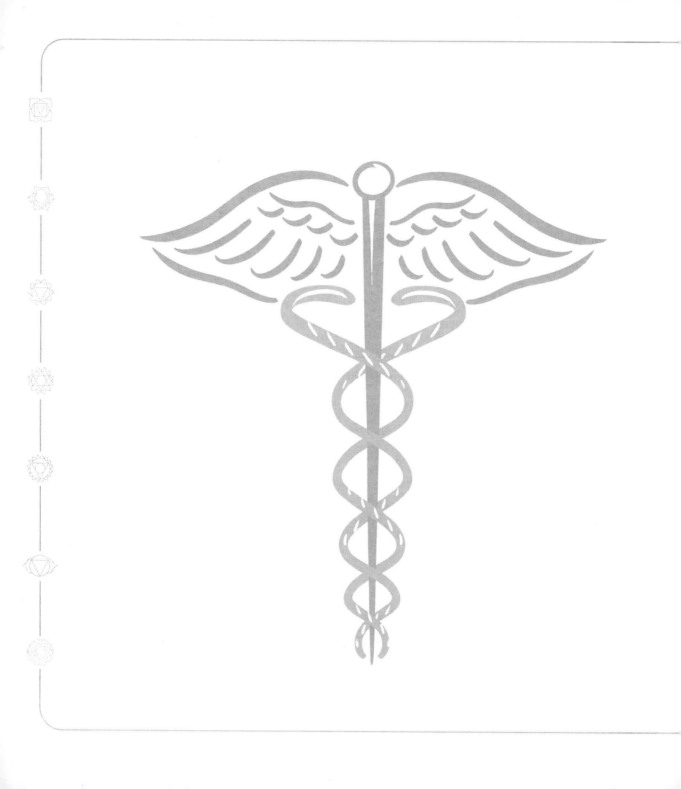

part three

The Meditations
of Kundalini Yoga

Meditations

Meditation in Kundalini Yoga is a *harnessing* and a *guiding* of energy through the psyche to the parts of ourselves that may need healing. It is an applied science that uses breath, mantra, mudra and numerological timings. All of these 'forms' will take you to the ultimate reality, to know the Self.

In meditation we are tweaking and adjusting aspects of ourselves within the astral level. It is at this dimension that permanent work can be done. The astral realm is the subtle playground where we can visit and 'update' old beliefs, attitudes, patterns and behavioural traits that no longer serve us.

Meditation clears the subconscious mind, it releases fears and issues that hold us back from being our true selves. It quietens the internal noise and takes us to a place of ultimate peace and surrender. Daily practice of meditation will change your life dramatically.

To achieve the most benefit from meditation, it has become known that practising a meditation for 40-day periods can bring about permanent change. The number 40 has a mystique attached to it. It is a number that has been used in ancient times to adjust traits within mankind. Jesus spent 40 days in the wilderness, 40 days and 40 nights were spent on the Ark, it took Moses 40 years to take his people through the desert and only at the age of 40 can a man begin to study the Kabbalah within Jewish culture.

It is understood that it takes 40 days to break a habit or pattern. To achieve these results you will have to commit to a daily meditation for 40 days. If you miss a day, you will have to start again at day one. Keep a diary to record all that begins to happen to you and to also keep track of what day you are on.

When you are in meditation you become a gateway for cosmic energy. The vibration of the Cosmos breaks through the antenna (the mudra) and into the gateway (the body) and merges into the blueprint that awakens the latent being. The wounds within are healed when you meditate. If you don't meditate the pain will come up in another area in your life. We tend to avoid meditation because of non-commitment. We feel that we do not have the time, we are too busy. To meditate is to listen to your Self. Are you really too busy to listen to your inner voice? Is there really no time to devote to hearing the words of your highest truth?

To begin with it may be challenging to meditate, as many thoughts and images will come up before you as your mind begins to release its turmoil. Every thought contains your own essence, even the really negative ones. Usually we cannot deal with these negative thoughts, so we decide to bury them. When in meditation they come up, we allow them, with no judgement, we become 'the watcher' the presence behind the thinking. As the thought is released so our Soul is cleansed.

Timings

In Kundalini Yoga there is a significant amount of importance placed upon timings and the number of repetitions in an exercise. This all goes back to sacred numerology, and the cosmic vibration of numbers. The duration of time held in meditation varies from 3, 11, 31 and 62 minutes.

Three Minutes

A posture or meditation held for three minutes will be working on the aura. It takes three minutes for one blood cell to leave the heart, travel through the body and come back to the heart again. Therefore, within three minutes the whole body will receive the information contained within the meditation or posture. Within that blood cell, there will be the vibration or the mantra, the focus of the exercise, the chemical adjustments of the breathing pattern and the invocation of the mudra. When the whole of the physical body has received the message of the meditation, the aura will reflect simultaneously.

Three signifies the three aspects of us: Mind, Body and Spirit, and the three aspects of God: to create, to sustain and to dissolve.

Eleven Minutes

Many meditations are for the duration of 11 minutes when we first begin practice. It takes this amount of time to stimulate the glandular system. Therefore, when holding the meditation for this time we have now moved to working on the glands. As we now know, the glandular system is responsible for a state of well-being, how we feel inside. With the release of certain hormones we perceive a sense of happiness, vitality and completeness. When the levels are depleted there will be feelings of sluggishness, loss of life and irritability. When the glandular system is finely tuned, all glands will be omitting the correct levels of hormones and the person will be in a state of emotional balance and stability. Therefore, when working with the number 11, we are working on the emotional bodies. In numerology, the number 11 breaks into one plus one equals two. Two is known to vibrate the energy of the Moon, which is always connected to the emotional realms, as the Moon waxes and wanes, so do our emotions.

Thirty-one Minutes

Three plus one equals four. Four is the number for stability, solidity and the base. In numerology we say that four represents Man. It is our structure and our solidity. When in meditation for 31 minutes we will be working on the nervous system. It is known that it takes 31 minutes to stimulate the three nervous systems within the body. The nervous system is responsible for our stamina, endurance and our capability to withstand the many challenges that life may throw our way. The nervous system will make us strong in the moment when the hurricane is all around us.

Sixty-two Minutes

Six plus two equals eight. Eight is the number for Infinity. When you draw the number eight there is no end, you can carry on forever following the shape of eight. This number has always been associated with 'the never ending'. When working with 62 minutes you will begin to stimulate the frontal brain. This, in turn, will stimulate the pineal and pituitary glands in the head.

Within this amount of time, you would have worked through the physical body, the emotions, the mental realms and now be in communication with the aspects of the Divine within.

It is these two glands that are known as the gateway to our higher consciousness. Through their secretions our consciousness is elevated to a level far beyond our normal everyday human perspective.

Yogi Bhajan has stated that within 62 minutes, you will begin to see God within everything.

Two and a Half Hours

Traditionally, this is the longest period of time in Kundalini yoga that we meditate as a prescribed time duration. Two and a half hours, breaks into 150 minutes. One plus five plus zero equals six. Six is the number that corresponds with the planet Venus, the energy of Love. When working with two and a half hours we begin to tap into the Love of God. This love is known as Bhakti, which translates as 'devotion'. Within this love is the gift of the Siddis. The Siddis are the magical powers attained through yoga. There are very secretive, but very real. In India you can see many demonstrations of various Siddis, such as levitation, manifestation of objects and being able to be in many places at the same time. When you get to this stage in the practice it can be where you trip up. To attain a magical power is not the goal, but a gift along the way.

Turbulent Times

A Meditation for Transformation

Now is the time when we begin to see chaos, fear and frustration in ourselves and in our environment. People are starting to go crazy, our nervous systems are beginning to fail and it looks as if the dark clouds are coming…

If you cannot help your neighbour in any other way, show them this meditation. Tape their hands together if you have to! But if you have mastered this meditation, just standing in your presence will lift the chaos from those around you. To master this kriya, practise for 120 days. That is the shortest possible time; it may take up to 40 years. Only sincere and earnest practice will bring forth the gifts of:

1. When you speak: the power of full understanding and listening will be given to the person you are speaking to.
2. Whatever you say, you will remember.
3. What you say shall be remembered by all who hear you.

You will begin to feel many things as you practise. Vast horizons will open up as you come to experience the truth…

YOGI BHAJAN

1. Easy Pose: Place your hands in fists at your diaphragm and touch the knuckles of the Saturn (middle) fingers. Extend the Jupiter (first) fingers away from the body and allow the pads at the end of the fingers to touch. Extend your thumbs back as far as you can, the thumbs are touching from the last knuckle to the tip. The mudra is held at the diaphragm and is touching the body.

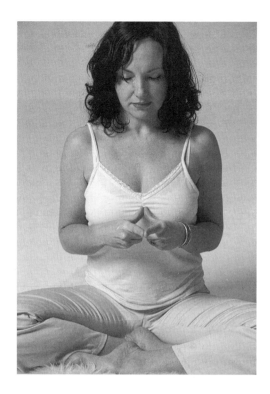

Inhale deeply into the diaphragm and begin to chant 'Wahe Guru' 40 times on one breath. When you run out of breath s stop chanting and begin again. You can begin by chanting 16 or 24 times as you build up to 40. 'Wahe Guru' should be chanted in three parts: Wa – Infinite, He – thou and Guru – the Self. The three-beat rhythm is very important.

Continue for 10–15 minutes. 31 minutes is a good time to practise this meditation.

Clearing the Past

*This meditation brings stress relief and clears the old emotions from the past.
This is especially beneficial to practise when dealing with painful relationships
and past family issues.*

HARIJOT KAUR KHALSA

1. Easy pose: Bend your elbows and bring
   your palms to the centre of your chest.
   Touch opposite fingers and thumbs to
   form a diamond with the hands. There is
   space between the palms and the mudra
   is points up. Stare at the tip of your nose
   and breathe four times per minute:
   Inhale five seconds, hold five seconds,
   exhale five seconds. Continue for 11
   minutes.

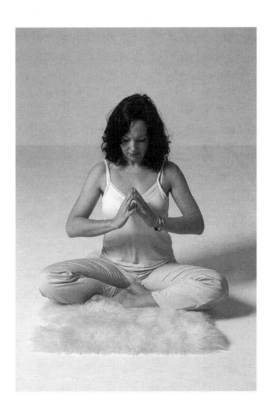

Meditation for Nerves of Steel

This meditation will give you a steady and strong endurance for when the going gets tough. It will protect you from being irrational and reactive.

SIRI DATTA

This meditation was given to us from Yogi Bhajan to 'prepare us for the grey period of the planet and to bring mental balance'.

1. Easy Pose: Bend your right arm and hold your right hand at ear level. Bring your thumb tip to the Sun (ring) finger. Place the left hand in your lap with the thumb tip touching the Mercury (little) finger. For women – please reverse both hand positions. Keep the posture steady and the spine straight.

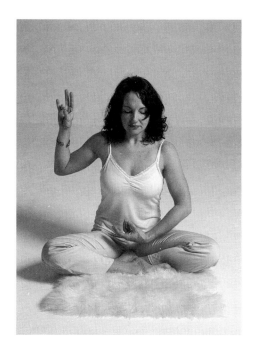

   The eyes are one-tenth open and you are breathing long and deep through the nose.

   You can begin practice for 11 minutes, but work up to 31 minutes. To end the meditation, inhale deeply, open the fingers, raise the arms overhead and shake them rapidly for a few minutes. Then relax.

Opening the Heart to Christ Consciousness

Smiling Buddha Kriya

Historically, this is an outstanding kriya. It was practised by both Buddha and Christ. The Great Brahman who taught Buddha this kriya found him nearly starved to death. Buddha was unable to walk after his 40-day fast under the fig tree. He began eating slowly and the great Brahman fed him and massaged him. When Buddha finally began to smile again, the Brahman gave him this one kriya to practise. Jesus also learned this during his travels. It was the first of many that he practised. If you love a man as great as he, it is important that you practise what he practised in order to achieve his state of consciousness. You will have probably seen this mudra in paintings and statues. It is a gesture and exercise of happiness and it opens the flow of energy into the Heart Centre. Do not learn it to be a Buddha or a Christ, learn it to be yourself. Master the technique and experience the state that it brings. Then share it by creating beauty and peace around you.

GURURATTAN KAUR KHALSA

1. Easy Pose: Bend the third and little fingers into the palm and lock them down with the thumb. Keep the first and second fingers extended. The fingers should be straight and the palms facing forwards. Elbows are bent and pressed back and the chest is pressed forwards. Make sure that there is a 30-degree angle between the upper and lower arms. Close the eyes and concentrate at the Brow Point and mentally chant:

SA TA NA MA

Sa – Infinity
Ta – Life
Na – Death
Ma – Rebirth

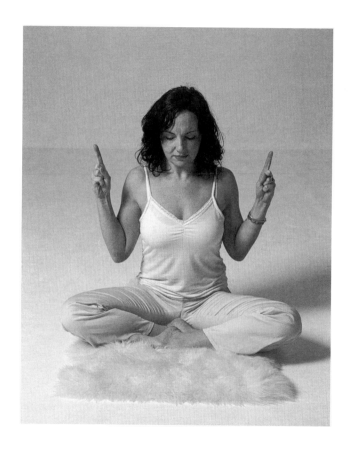

Continue for 11 minutes. To finish, inhale deeply, hold the breath 10 seconds, and exhale. As you exhale, open and close the fists rapidly several times. Relax.

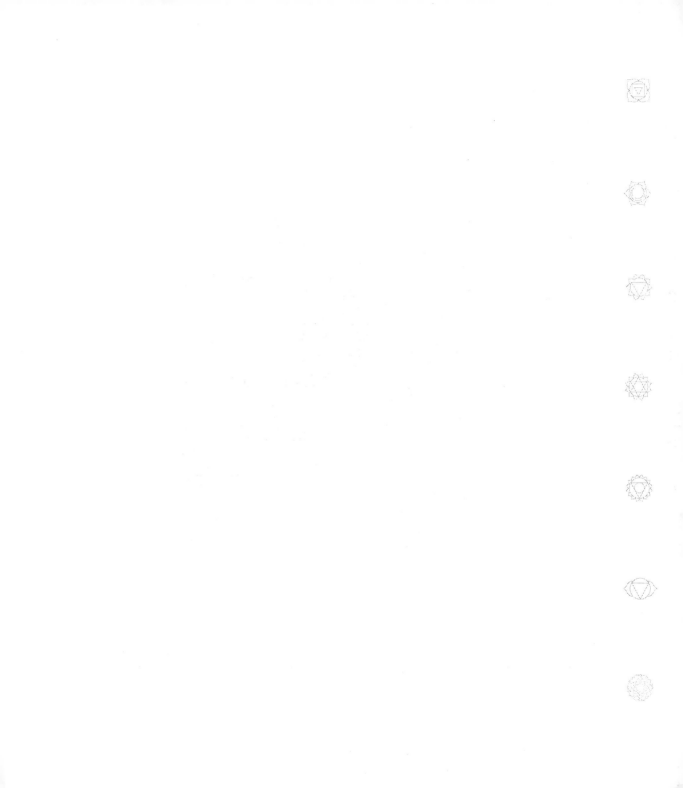

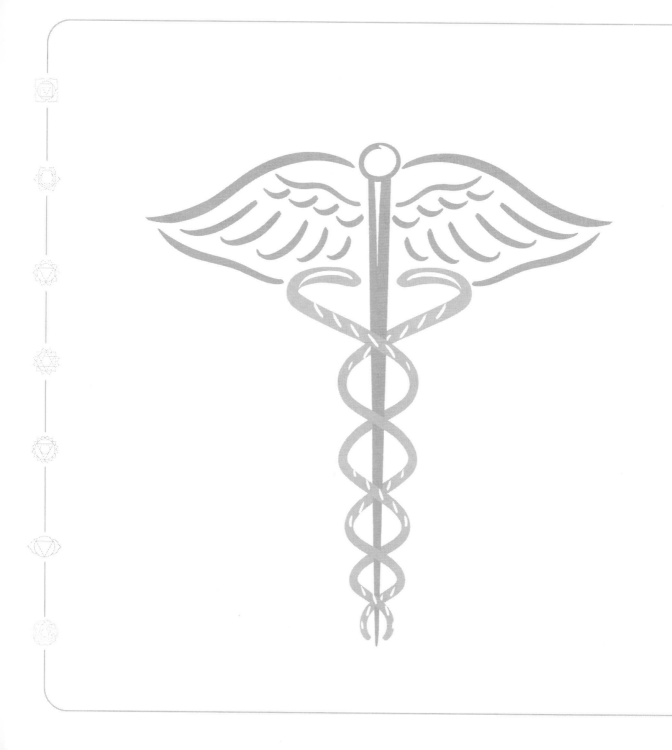

part five

Ancient Answers for Modern Living

Modern Day Issues

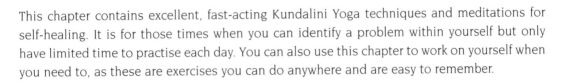

This chapter contains excellent, fast-acting Kundalini Yoga techniques and meditations for self-healing. It is for those times when you can identify a problem within yourself but only have limited time to practise each day. You can also use this chapter to work on yourself when you need to, as these are exercises you can do anywhere and are easy to remember.

Use these techniques as the necessary tools to maintain a healthy body and to help correct specific physical and mental problems.

It is important to keep in mind that yoga is only one aspect of self-healing. These techniques alone do not carry absolute confirmation that they will cure, heal or prevent any condition. If your problems are severe consult your doctor. Since lifestyle has a significant influence on health, the yogic concept of a healthy lifestyle is described in the last section (*see page* 203).

As modern health-care specialists are beginning to acknowledge, by far the most effective way to treat disease is to prevent it from occurring in the first place. While all yoga has the effect of boosting health, some exercises and meditations are very specific in their disease-prevention and therapeutic effects. If you detect illness coming on, these are excellent kriyas to practise to dissolve the effect.

Key areas of the body first need to be looked at to attain a vital understanding of the body and its state of well-being. We need to become aware of our body's tell-tale signs of imbalance.

Shoulders

Stiffness in the shoulders is a key sign to look out for as this has harmful effects on the well-being of the body. It is stated in *The Yellow Emperor's Classic of Internal Medicine* (written over 4,000 years ago) that the wind and cold enter the pores of the skin around the shoulderblades. It is important to keep this area flexible and resilient. In Ancient India, as well as China, it was understood that stiffness in the shoulderblades was considered to contribute to illness. There was a practice in these ancient times whereby a person would swing a thick branch, or club, back and forth to break down the tension in this area.

Feet

The feet are a strong centre for Pranic and electromagnetic field activity. Also, nerve endings in the feet reach every part of the body and affect the health of the body as a whole. That is why foot care is vital to good health. A natural way to take care of feet is to walk bare-foot. This will stimulate and massage them. But walking on concrete or hard surfaces is actually not so good, as it causes crystals and calluses to form. Be aware of your footwear, especially high heels, as they can cause the feet to become deformed and throw the spine and pelvis out of alignment. Because of their sensitivity and special relationship to the rest of the body, the feet can tell you a lot about the health of your body as a whole. A pain in the foot that is not related to direct injury can indicate that the body is about to become ill. Foot massage on that point is an excellent form of preventative care.

Lungs

In a physical sense, the lungs supply oxygen to the blood and life force, or Prana, to the body. Air pollution, smoking and incorrect breathing hinder this health-giving process. Smoking is our choice. If you would like to stop smoking, practise the 'Addiction Meditation' (*see page* 191). Just as important is the question of correct breathing. The average person breathes about 15 times per minute, while a practised yogi breathes about eight times per minute. To develop a truly meditative mind you will need to reduce the breaths to four times per minute.

Without sustained breath, you will not reach the deeper parts of the lungs. As a result, the blood is improperly purified. This leads to a thickening of the arteries and clogged capillaries. The magnetic field is diminished, the nerves become weak, and the body wears out and loses its resistance to disease. In India it is known that we all have a certain number of breaths to breathe in the course of life. It is a fact that those who breathe deeply are less prone to hypertension, heart disease, nervous tension, digestive disorders and high blood pressure.

If you practise the following breathing exercises the entire blood supply will be cleansed several times: ten minutes of left-hand nostril breathing, followed by ten minutes of right-hand nostril breathing, ten minutes of long, deep breathing through both nostrils and ten minutes of Breath of Fire (*see page* 61).

Liver

A healthy liver is essential to overall well-being. The liver manufactures, cleanses and balances the ingredients of the blood. Its malfunction causes death. Meats, oily foods, eggs, poorly cooked or rancid foods, chemicals and preservatives all tax the liver. Alcohol intake and over-eating are the most destructive things we can do to the liver. Cleansing juice diets will help rebuild and detoxify an abused liver. See the section on diet (*see page* 210) for juice diets and fasting.

Navel Point

Masters of the martial arts have known for centuries about the unique nature of the Navel Point as the centre for power and balance in the body. It is the Navel Centre, which ensures that the 72,000 nerves and arteries that spread over the entire body perform their assigned tasks. We may take precautions to keep the body free of disease. We feed it, exercise it, treat it with medicine, but if the Navel Point is off-balance, all these efforts will be in vain. You can see if your Navel Point is off by doing the following experiment. Lie down on your back and press the thumb and fingers of one hand firmly into the navel. Somewhere near the navel you will feel a strong pulse. If this pulse is exactly at the navel, it is said that the Navel Point is centred. This indicates that your state of health is good. Displacement of the navel pulse in an upward position can be associated with constipation, acid blood, heart disease and general irritation. A displacement downwards causes colic pain and bad dreams. Fortunately simple exercises are available to centre the navel. One such exercise is Stretch Pose (*see page* 111). Daily practice of Stretch Pose will bring the navel back into balance. As this happens, you should feel renewed poise, power and inner strength.

Stress Reduction

Stress is the number-one killer in the Western world, according to medical studies. It is the cause of heart failure, drug abuse and many other diseases. The most common remedy for stress is to treat the symptoms with tranquillizers, alcohol and tobacco or to hide them in chronic television-viewing or overeating. Stimulation is then required, such as coffee, cigarettes and drugs to replace the depleted energy. This is like driving the car with one foot on the accelerator and the other on the brake. This is what we are doing to the heart and adrenal glands.

Another approach to stress reduction is offered by professional therapists and counsellors. These do give temporary relief, but they can fail to deliver long-term results. This is because they are not dealing with the longing of the human spirit to be in harmony with the rest of the being. A permanent and successful treatment for stress must operate in a metaphysical framework. For it is only when we realize the vastness of our unlimited and divine identity that we can begin to find inner peace and happiness. In these pages are techniques to work on stress and tension, designed to bring the wholeness of the human being back together.

Addiction

This meditation is excellent for everyone, but particularly effective for rehabilitation efforts in drug dependence, mental illness and phobic conditions. It also works on subconscious addictions, which lead us to insecure or neurotic behaviour patterns. In modern culture, the imbalance is epidemic. If we are not addicted to smoking, overeating, drugs or drinking, then we are addicted subconsciously to acceptance, advancement, rejection or emotional love. All these lead us to insecure and neurotic behaviour.

The pressure exerted by the thumbs triggers a rhythmic reflex current into the central brain. This current activates the brain area directly underneath the stem of the pineal gland. If there is an imbalance in this area it will make mental and physical addictions seem unbreakable.

1. Easy Pose: With a straight spine, make sure that the lowest six vertebrae are pushed forwards. Make fists of your hands. Extend the thumbs out and place them on your temples in the niche where they fit and you feel a pulse. Lock your back molars and keep your lips closed. Vibrate the jaw muscles by alternating the pressure on the molars. A muscle will move in rhythm under your thumbs as you apply a firm pressure.

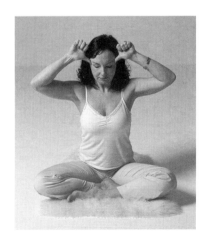

2. Keep your eyes closed. Look to the Third Eye Point and mentally chant the mantra 'Sa Ta Na Ma'.

3. Continue for five to seven minutes. The time may be extended to 20–31 minutes with practice.

Arthritis

This exercise is also very effective for constipation and improving eyesight.

Cold showers are excellent for arthritis. Be sure to rub oil into your body first. Do not precede or end your shower with warm water. Early in the morning get up and rub almond oil into your body until it becomes red, then take a cold shower. (*See Part 6, Beauty section, page* 229). Glucosamine Sulphate is an excellent supplement for arthritis. This mineral is usually found in shellfish.

1. Sit down with your legs spread as wide apart as possible. Inhale up and stretch the spine, exhale over, bringing your forehead as close to the floor as possible. Reach to hold on to your heels, ankles or shins. Be aware of your spine bending from the hips. Make sure your legs stay straight, with the backs of your knees on the floor. Stay bending forwards and breathe normally through your nose. Continue for one to three minutes.

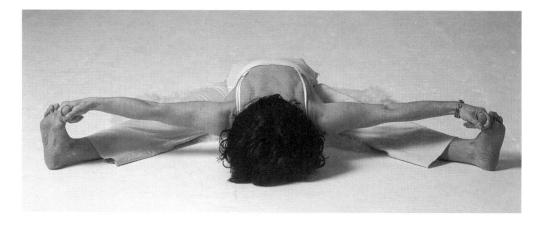

Asthma

This exercise is said to make asthma fly away like a crow at the clap of your hands!

1. Stand up with your heels together, but with your feet slightly angled outwards to give you balance. Arms are overhead and your palms held together by interlocking the thumbs. Inhale up and stretch your entire spine and arms and then lean back as far as possible and do Breath of Fire for one to three minutes. To avoid falling, you could bend back against the back of a sofa or you could get someone to support you. You must bend back as far as possible. Keep your arms straight, with your pelvis pushed forwards. Drop your head and keep your eyes closed. Do not allow your spine to collapse. Keep stretching up and back. Breathe as long and deep as you can.

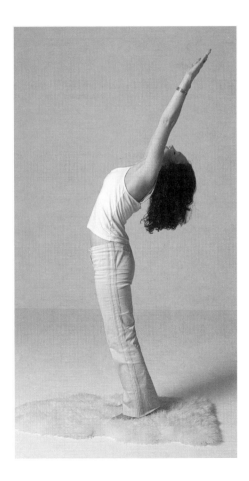

Blood Pressure

High Blood Pressure

Breathing through the left nostril stimulates the 'Moon' functions of the body. When you have a lot of lunar energy you will be relaxed, calm and level-headed. Lunar energy keeps the body cool, sensitive and intuitive. The breath flows mainly through one nostril at any one time. The flow of breath switches from one nostril to the other every two and a half hours throughout the day. You can automatically channel this flow to your left nostril by holding your left hand under your right armpit, with your right arm pressing down on your left hand slightly. Try it!

1. Easy Pose: Use the thumb of your right hand to block your right nostril. Point the fingers of your right hand straight up. Do Breath of Fire through your left nostril while pumping your navel in and out. The more you pull your abdomen in and push it out again, the more effective this kriya will be. Continue for one to three minutes. For long-standing problems of high blood pressure, carry out daily practice of 40 minutes of normal left-nostril breathing (without Breath of Fire or pumping the stomach).

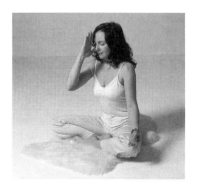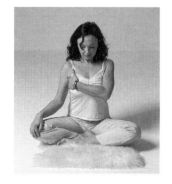

Low Blood Pressure

Breathing through your right nostril stimulates the 'Sun' functions of the body. When you have a lot of Sun energy you will find that you do not get cold, you are energetic, extroverted and enthusiastic. It is the energy of purification and it is this energy that holds the weight down. It aids digestion, makes the mind clear, analytical and action-orientated.

By reversing the above exercise, you will be working on balancing low blood pressure. Again, with long-standing problems of low blood pressure, you should practise 40 minutes of normal right-nostril breathing daily.

Drug Damage

To repair nerve damage due to the misuse of drugs, do this exercise once a day for 40 days. Also, drink golden milk during this time.

To make golden milk: Boil ⅛ of a teaspoon of turmeric in a cup of water for about eight minutes, until it forms a thick paste. Meanwhile, pour 225 ml (8 fl oz) of milk into a pan and bring to the boil. After the milk has boiled then add 1 teaspoon of almond oil. It is rendered unhealthy if you mix the oil and milk together during the boiling process. Combine the two mixtures and add honey to taste.

1. Cat Cow: Get on to your hands and knees. Make sure that your knees are a hips'-width apart and that your palms are underneath your shoulders, the same distance apart. Your toes are flat on the floor and your lower legs are parallel. Begin flexing your spine up and down. Inhale as the spine arches up, sticking your tailbone up, dipping your chest and lifting up with the head and shoulders. When you inhale, really open up your throat as you lift your head back. Keep your posture steady until you have breathed in all you can. As you exhale, round off your spine, bringing your chin to your chest. You can press up with your arms to make sure your spine is lifted as you exhale. Really concentrate on bringing your head as close to your thighs as possible. Hold this posture until you have fully breathed out and then inhale up again. Continue for three minutes.

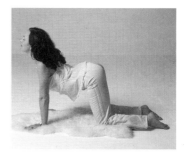

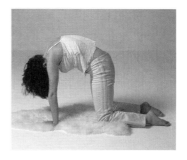

Depression

This meditation is an antidote to depression. You will find that if you do it properly it will totally recharge you. It will give you the capacity to deal with life well.

1. Easy Pose: Extend your arms straight out in front, parallel to the floor. Close your right hand into a fist. Wrap the fingers of your left hand around the right-hand fist. Let the bases of your palms touch. Your thumbs are close together and are pulled straight up. Your eyes are focused on your thumbs. Inhale slowly for five seconds (do not hold the breath in); exhale slowly for five seconds; hold the breath out for 15 seconds. Continue like this for three to five minutes, and work up to 11 minutes. Make sure your arms stay parallel and your elbows remain straight. Build up the time slowly. With practice you will be able to hold the breath out for one minute. However, take care not to hold the breath until the point of dizziness or nausea.

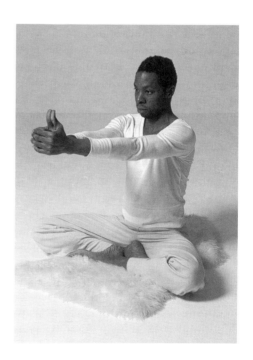

Insomnia

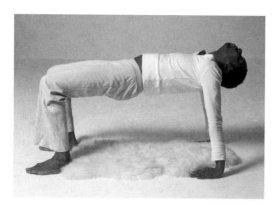
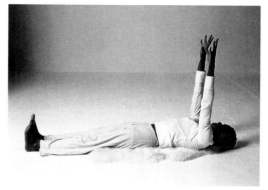

1. Bridge Pose: Lie on your back. From this position, bend your knees and lift up on to all-fours. Place your palms under your shoulders and your feet underneath your knees. Keep your feet square, and make sure your fingers point towards the feet. They too should be square and the same distance apart as your shoulders. Keep your body in a straight line: your shoulders, hips and knees should be in line with each other. Your head is parallel to the ceiling. Do Breath of Fire for 5–20 minutes. Then inhale completely, exhale and relax down onto your back again.

2. Corpse Pose: Inhale completely. Reaching up with your arms, make sure your hands are open and stretching towards the ceiling. Hold your breath in as you make fists of your hands, and very very slowly pull your fists towards your chest. There must be so much tension in your arms and hands that they shake. Imagine that you are pulling a very heavy weight towards you. When your fists reach your chest, exhale. Relax.

Mental Fatigue

You should only do this meditation when you can relax afterwards. Done correctly, it is very effective against 'brain drain'. It imparts a balanced mental state and can give you an unimaginable amount of powerful energy.

1. Easy Pose: With a straight spine, extend your Sun (fourth) fingers and place them together. Interlock the rest of your fingers and place your right thumb over the top of your left. Hold this mudra a short distance away from your diaphragm, at a 60-degree angle upwards. Close your eyes. Inhale deeply and powerfully. Exhale as you chant out loud the mantra 'ong'. Keep your mouth open, but let all the air flow through your nose as you chant. The sound will be far back and up in the upper palate. Keep the sound going until you run out of breath. Continue for three minutes. The power of this chant, when correctly done, has to be experienced to be believed. Only five repetitions are needed to totally elevate the consciousness.

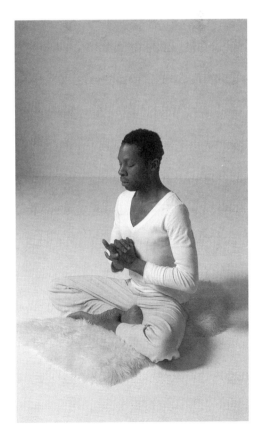

Premenstrual Tension

1. Standing, with your knees and heels together, have your feet flat on the floor, but slightly angled outwards. Raise your arms straight up overhead; bring the sides of your upper arms close to your ears, with the palms facing forwards. Your thumbs can be locked together. Keeping your legs straight, bend back from the base of the spine 20 degrees, push forwards with the hips and open up your ribs and breastbone. The head, spine and arms form an unbroken curve with your arms in line with your ears. Hold this posture with long, deep, gentle breathing for two minutes.

2. From this position, very slowly bend over as far as possible, keeping your arms straight and close to your ears. Inhale deeply and while the breath is being held begin to pump the Navel Point. Then exhale, and continue pumping the navel on the exhaled breath. Inhale again. Continue pumping your navel on the inhale and exhale for two further minutes.

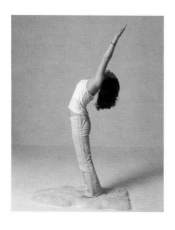 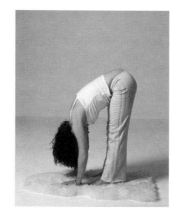

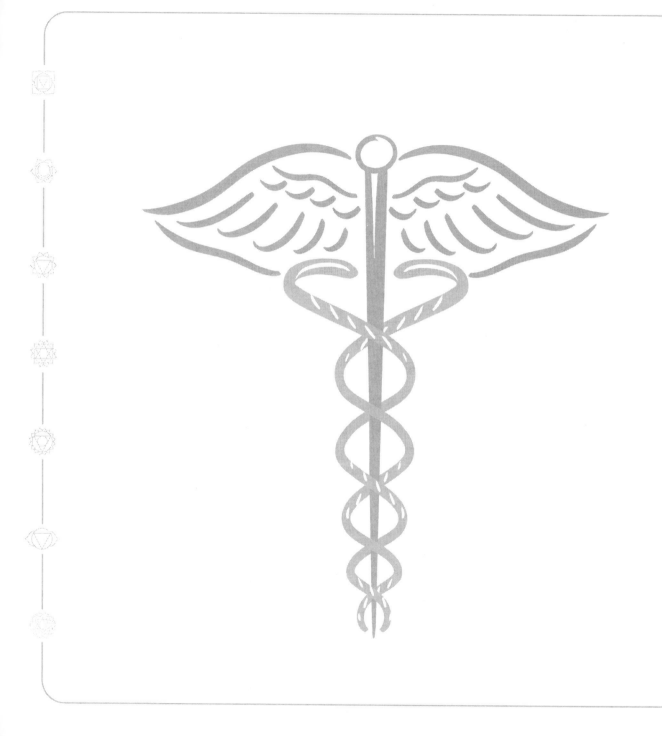

part six

The Yogic Lifestyle

Yogic Lifestyle

Compiled by the Sage Patanjali in the Yoga Sutras, the Eight Limbs are a progressive series of steps or disciplines that give a clear path on how to achieve a yogic lifestyle.

The steps are:

- Yamas (universal ethical principles)
- Niyamas (rules of personal conduct)
- Asanas (postures)
- Pranayama (breathing exercises)
- Pratyahara (control of the senses)
- Dharana (concentration of the mind)
- Dhyana (meditation)
- Samadhi (enlightenment)

The yamas are divided into five moral codes, aimed at transcending the lower nature of ourselves: non-violence, truthfulness, non-stealing, moderation in all things and non-possessiveness.

The niyamas are also divided into five: purity, contentment, austerity, study of sacred texts and living in awareness of the Divine.

Pratyahara means drawing of the senses inwards in order to still the mind, in preparation for Dhyana, or meditation, cultimating in Samadhi, or Enlightenment.

The Five Principles

By closely observing the lifestyles and needs of people in the West, Swami Vishu Devananda from the Sivananda yoga discipline has synthesized the ancient wisdom of yoga into five basic principles that can be easily incorporated into your everyday lifestyle.

- **Proper Relaxation** releases tension in the muscles and rests the whole system, leaving you as refreshed as if you had had a good night's sleep.
- **Proper Exercise** is given by the yoga postures, which work systematically on all parts of the body, mind and spirit.
- **Proper Breathing** means breathing deeply and rhythmically, making full use of your lungs to increase your intake of oxygen. This gives you complete control over your flow of Prana; the life force, conserved in the chakras.
- **Proper Diet** is one that is nourishing and well balanced, based on natural foods. It keeps the body light and supple and the mind calm, giving a high resistance to disease.
- **Positive Thinking and Meditation** helps you to remove negative thoughts and still the mind, ultimately transcending all thoughts.

There are two other areas I would add to these everyday principles and they are:

- **Proper Preparation** of the body by following a daily routine.

There is a very simple daily routine that Yogi Bhajan has given the West to practise every day to prepare for the day ahead. The first step is:

○ Wake yourself up by subconsciously telling yourself what time you want to get up. Leaping out of bed when the alarm goes off damages your nervous system. Your sub-conscious mind will easily wake you at exactly what time you please.
○ Stretching while still in bed. Take a few deep breaths to stretch out the whole spine before you get up.
○ Cat Stretch: Bend one knee to your chest and stretch over to the opposite side, stretching and twisting your spine. This is good for your circulation and adjusts the electromagnetic field to its balance point.

- Massage your face. Massage your forehead from the centre out to the temples and down both sides of the face towards your chin. Begin to massage your nose and ears, squeezing your nostrils and earlobes.
- Stretch Pose: Lying on your back with your legs straight, bring your heels together and lift your head and heels 15 cm (6 in) off the bed. Eyes open, focusing on your toes. Hold the position for one minute with Breath of Fire *(see pranayama section, page 57)*. Hold your arms straight at your sides, palms facing each other above your thighs.
- Bring your knees to your chest and clasp your hands around your knees. Relax in this posture. Lift your head to your knees and begin Breath of Fire for 30 seconds. This stimulates the Apana (out-going life force) and elimination.
- Rest the heart. In this same position, roll over on to your right side and rest for a minute or two. This posture strengthens the heart.
- Walk barefoot to the bathroom. It is better to be barefoot, so that your body can discharge any excess electromagnetic energy that you have accumulated overnight.
- Toileting. When you go to the toilet first thing in the morning, you can verify how your digestion system is working. If your stools float, that is a good sign. It means you have taken all the food value from whatever you ingested the day before. If your stool sinks, something is wrong with your diet or your digestive system, probably both. The colour of your urine should not be darker than gold.
- Brush your tongue. It is very important to brush the root of your tongue. During the night your mouth will start to produce bacteria and we need to get rid of this toxic accumulation. Unless we get rid of it, with our first mouthful of tea in the morning, we swallow it back down into the system. To avoid self-poisoning, brush the root of your tongue, until you gag. Then you know you have hit the spot. Another benefit of gagging is that the water you produce in your eyes is very beneficial for helping to avoid cataracts and to improve your eyesight.
- Take a cold shower. Before you get under the shower, massage your skin all over with almond oil. This will replace any minerals that you may have lost through your skin, plus it keeps the skin soft and supple. This is called hydrotherapy. It strengthens your entire nervous system, does wonders for your circulation and stimulates your glandular system. Go under the water four times, continuously massaging your body until you no longer feel cold.

- **Proper Sleep,** of which there are six steps:

  o Make sure you have carried out some strenuous exercise during the day so that your Physical Body is ready to rest. Everyone needs to exercise until they sweat every day.
  o Do not eat a heavy meal before bedtime. You need the digestive system to slow down. Eat at least four hours before you go to bed.
  o Brush your teeth and tongue to get rid of any bacteria.
  o Do not go to bed thirsty. Drink at least one or two glasses of water before you go to sleep. If you go to bed thirsty, your body will be dehydrated and that disturbs the mind, preventing proper rest, even causing bad dreams.
  o Run some cold water over your feet, and then dry them vigorously with a towel. This will stimulate the 72,000 nerve endings in the sole of each foot, and get the nervous system ready for sleep.
  o Either read something inspirational, meditate, play some beautiful music and then let go into deep relaxation. As thoughts come up, let them go.

Four Simple Steps to Deep Sleep

  o Lie on your stomach and turn your head so that your right cheek is on the pillow. This will free up your left nostril to bring in cooling, soothing and calming energy.
  o Start long, deep breathing through your nose, keeping your mouth closed.
  o After a few long deep breaths use your arm or hand to completely block off your right nostril. Continue breathing through your left nostril.
  o When you feel yourself starting to get drowsy, turn over on to your back, or however you wish to sleep. It is better for your heart and digestion to sleep on your right side. Continue long, deep breathing.

As soon as your breath becomes regular and slow, you will go quickly through the preliminary stages of sleep and almost immediately reach the deep dreamless sleep state, avoiding the energy-draining dream state. Another sleep-enhancer is to sprinkle a few drops of lavender oil on to your pillow.

H.H. Sri Swami Sivananda was another great Yogi and sage who devoted his life to the service of humanity and the study of Vedanta. His prescription for a spiritual life is summed up in six simple commands:

- Serve
- Love
- Give
- Purify
- Meditate
- Realize

Foods that Heal

Food is the medicine that creates essential energy in the body and essential rest that restores equilibrium. There are two types of food, nutritious and sustaining. Nutritious foods are those that give your body strength, endurance and stamina. Sustaining foods are those that heal the body, maintain the internal systems and keep the body in balance. Apart from being nutritious and sustaining, food should also be balanced. Balanced food is that which can be digested without drawing on your health. There are many types of food, but the food that sustains you will bring you the greater joy. You do not grow old with years, you grow old with food.

This is based on the traditional art of Ayurveda. There are lots of foods available to us today that are not part of the original Ayurveda tradition. In this chapter there is nothing that is not part of this traditional method. The foods that are mentioned in this section, are foods that have benefited certain conditions. These are not tried-and-tested means. Please note that a lengthy fast should never be undertaken without professional supervision.

Alcoholism

The problem in the alcoholic is the breakdown in the kidney, adrenal and liver systems. Massage the points on the feet that relate to those organs. An ancient dietary cure for alcoholism is to eat only beetroot and Brewer's Yeast for three days. Even if you are not hungry, you must eat it. Juices are very helpful, especially grapefruit juice. Another juice alternative is to drink carrot and celery juice every two hours. The ratio is 1:3 and 3:1 alternately. Large doses of the B vitamins, in particular pantothenic acid, is very helpful. Vitamin C is very useful to alcoholics.

Cleansing

Thirty-Day Diet

If you are eager to begin a distinct improvement to your health, then try a special diet of eating just fruits, nuts and vegetables for 30 days. This diet is used in India when the person looks old and the body is wearing out. It cleans the system and revitalizes the body. After 30 days, eat milk products. The best time to start this diet is in the spring, summer and autumn, when the weather is warm and these foods are available fresh. This is a build-up diet that will pave the way for the ideal yogic diet.

Broccoli Fast

For 30 days eat only one green vegetable; broccoli is recommended. This is a good diet for cleansing and very helpful in meditation. This diet needs to be broken with one day of lemon juice, water and honey.

Lettuce Fast

This is a week-long lettuce fast for detoxification. You can add a dressing of broth powder (dehydrated vegetables; available from most health stores) and some olive (or almond) oil. Tear the lettuce leaves by hand rather than using a knife. For breakfast have orange juice, for lunch have lettuce and for dinner have birch leaf tea with some honey. If you get really hungry in the evening, have some fruit.

Mung Beans and Rice

This is a great cleansing diet. It is good for the kidneys and helps in deep meditation. This diet will work on the colon and digestive organs. For 30 days eat only mung beans and rice. You can also add many varieties of green vegetables. Eat fruit between meals when you like. Drink yogi tea. (*See the section on recipes, page* 000).

Raw Vegetable Juices

Raw vegetable juice, from organically grown vegetables, is the easiest way to ingest a high percentage of vitamins and minerals, which the body craves. These juices are very regenerative for the body, as it only takes 15 minutes for the juice to be totally assimilated into the body. You must not drink the juices, but 'eat' them, thoroughly chewing them and mixing them with saliva. Raw juice fasts are good for losing weight, detoxification and cleansing the cells, organs and tissues of the body.

Apples, garlic, grapes, milk, parsley, water and yoghurt have effective cleansing properties.

Apples

Apples are cleansing, however they are prepared.

Garlic

Eat three cloves of garlic, morning, noon and night to cure all sickness. Drink lots of water with the garlic. Try spreading raw garlic cloves on rice cakes.

Grapes

Grapes are a wonderful blood-purifier and builder. They are high in vitamin C, magnesium and potassium. A diet of grapes only has been used to detoxify the body, transform the blood stream and to overcome chronic diseases. Green grapes are good for a clear complexion.

Milk

Going on a milk fast is quite difficult, but it is reported that it can cure cancer. The scriptures tell us that blood poisoning, lymph gland problems or any impurity can be cured in five to six days by drinking milk that has been boiled with black peppercorns. Swallow them whole and leave the rest to God.

Parsley

Parsley is rich in minerals, especially calcium, potassium and sulphur. It is a good kidney cleanser, blood-builder and it controls the calcium in the body. Parsley juice is good for eliminating poisonous foods from the body.

Water

We all need to drink lots of water. Water keeps our system clean. The stomach is divided into four parts: one for food, one for water, one for air and one empty to let it work efficiently.

Yogurt

Home-made yogurt is a natural cleanser of the stomach and intestines. It neutralizes acidic conditions and enriches intestinal flora. Externally it makes the best shampoo and body cleanser.

Detoxification

This section is for people who have taken drugs and who want to detoxify their bodies. You will need to do at least these two fasts to remove all the drug deposits in the body.

Banana Fast

This diet removes drug deposits from the medulla. It must be started on the New Moon and continued for 14 days until the Full Moon. It is intended to build up worn tissues and adjusts the iron, sodium and potassium in the body. This diet takes away the sodium and replaces the calcium.

Breakfast: 1 cup of freshly squeezed orange juice with the pulp left in, and sweetened with honey. After one hour, eat three bananas. Chew thoroughly. This is very important. Be sure to eat the strings of white that cling to the banana. Immediately afterwards eat the contents of one cardamom pod. The cardamom turns the bananas into liquid and changes their effect in the digestive system.

Lunch: three bananas, followed by one cardamom pod.
Dinner: three bananas, followed by one cardamom pod.

This diet has its side-effects. You may feel weak from the lack of customary nervous stimulus. In that case take more orange juice and honey during the day. If constipation is the problem, increase the cardamom pods to a maximum of three at a time. Also, drink large amounts of hot water periodically. You can drink yogi tea with this diet. If you have a severe reaction to this diet, stop immediately.

The banana fast is not recommended for people who have not been on previous cleansing or purification diets.

On the fifteenth day of the Moon, you should take only lemon juice in warm water with honey. Then, for the next 28 days, you should go on the mung bean and rice diet. Do not have dairy products during these 28 days.

Beetroot Fast

This is a very heavy fast, not to be taken lightly at all. This level of liver-cleansing will be very intense, so caution will be needed. This fast is to remove drug deposits from the body. Keep eating beetroot and drinking beetroot juices until everything is red when you go to the toilet, and then continue until it is no longer red.

Colds and Infections

To avoid colds, go on a warm-water-only diet for one day. Mondays or Thursdays are good for this diet. Water helps keeping the bowels moving. If you have a chest cold apply eucalyptus oil externally to the throat and chest area. Quinine, yogi tea and watermelon juice will help.

Quinine

Quinine comes from the cinchona tree. You should take five grains in a capsule if flu or a cold is coming on. It energizes the energy centres. Be sure to drink lots if milk, at least 225 ml (8 fl oz) after taking quinine.

Yogi Tea

Yogi tea is a mild stimulant and it also eliminates air pockets from the spine. A three-day yogi tea diet is great for flu or any kind of respiratory cold.

Watermelon Juice

This is highly cleansing and regulates the liver. It works with the kidneys to get them to secrete more efficiently, stops mucus formation and cools down the membranes within the kidneys. Try drinking watermelon juice instead of having a meal.

Vitamin C

Take vitamin C regularly if you have an infectious disease or are under heavy stress. 3 g (¼ oz) is very good to minimize the effects of smog and air in lightly polluted areas. When you take a high dosage of vitamin C (10 g (½ oz per day) and then you decide to come off it, you may well notice that you get a reaction known as 'rebound survey'. This is a vitamin C deficiency, when your body is used to receiving 10 g (½ oz) per day and suddenly you stop, you will experience a relative deficiency. Always taper off slowly over a few days or weeks, depending on how long you have been taking it.

Drug Abuse

Yogi therapy says that if a person is disturbed because of drug-taking, massage their feet with a mixture of almond oil and garlic juice. To restore the nerve centres damaged by drug abuse, drink Golden Milk (*see page* 227) every day for 40 days and practise the meditation on drug damage (*see page* 196). Pineapple juice gives energy and is good for a person on tranquillizers or who is drug-addicted.

Smoking

There are two things known in yogic therapy that help with giving up smoking: eat a packet of raisins every day and practise Vatskar Kriya. This is a breathing technique where you curl the tongue and drink air through the curled tongue as though you are sipping through a straw. You exhale through the nose. Continue until you feel a bitter taste on your tongue.

Energy

Use a wooden comb whenever you feel low in energy. Just comb your hair through with a wooden comb. It is like having an immediate energy shot. You could also try an energy drink to take away fatigue. Take 225 ml (8 fl oz) of cucumber juice, two tablespoons of liquid chlorophyll (water-soluble), two tablespoons of protein powder and two tablespoons of lecithin. Blend it all together and drink. Lecithin is the nectar of life.

Jalapeno Pancake Diet

This diet is guaranteed to make 'skinnies' lose weight. It is the most abundant way to increase energy.

Take equal parts of finely chopped ginger and cauliflower. Use one finely chopped jalapeno per pancake. Add ajwan seeds (oregano), crushed red chillies, black pepper, amino acids, equal parts bran and wholewheat flour (half a cup each per pancake works well). Mix with enough water to make a thick batter. Cook on a surface coated with lecithin so that the batter will not stick. Cook for 15 minutes per side. Eat two pancakes per day: one in the morning and one in the early evening. Have with one glass of skimmed milk.

Apples

Apples are blood cleansers and purifiers. They are high in sodium, potassium, magnesium and vitamins C and B. An apple in the morning will overcome any weakness in the body.

Bananas
Bananas are great energy foods.

Carrots
Carrots have vitamin C and calcium. They increase vitality.

Coconuts
Coconuts are known to be good for fatigue and general weakness.

Dates
Dates are a rich source of quick energy. They are easy to digest and they give heat to the whole body. They are good for undernourished people and for those with a hypoactive thyroid. Dates simmered in milk make a rebuilding energy drink.

Garlic
Garlic is an energy-giver; it does this by removing all pesticides from our food. One reason why people may be low in energy is because of these added toxins. One way to remove these toxins is to consume garlic either in the form of raw garlic or supplements.

Ginger
Ginger tea is particularly good for menstrual cramps and general fatigue. Boil four or five slices of fresh ginger root in three cups of water; add honey to taste and drink. This works directly on the fourth vertebra and lower back, and is therefore very beneficial for relief of backache. It is also very good for flu and colds.

Sesame Oil and Milk
Mix sesame oil with hot milk and drink before you go to bed. This will clear the system by

morning, leaving you very energetic after a few days' treatment.

Fasting

The best time to go on a fast is in the spring. It is the springtime when the new blood comes into the system and indeed any dietary precaution that you take on should be started in the springtime. Do not attempt a fast without preparing for it, and without the capacity to go through with it. Without preparation, a fast can actually damage your metabolism and energy rather than doing any good. You need to prepare by making sure the body is fit and well. Look at your days ahead by making sure that not too much is being asked of you physically. Ideally, when fasting you should be resting at home, getting the right amount of sleep and generally healing the body. It is not a good idea to fast while still carrying out a demanding everyday job. Plan your fast, making sure friends know that you are having quality time to yourself, take plenty of rest and make sure that you carry out yoga and meditation to cleanse the mind.

Mono-diets

A mono-diet for a woman should last for between five and ten days. If you plan to go on a mono-diet for more than 10 days, you should consult a specialist.

Fruit Fast

When the spring comes start a total fruit diet. This means just fruit, no juices. Do not mix the fruits, as they each have very precise actions. You cannot have one kind of fruit in the morning and then another in the afternoon and you cannot mix fruits in the same meal. Have one kind of fruit at a time.

Juice Fast

Juice is a good fast, but it is not good for the intestinal tract and it is not normally recommended. When fasting you have to be able to empty your bowels, and there is no substance in juice to form a stool. So you must carry out a juice fast with extreme caution and wisdom. It does, however, clean the lungs, liver, kidneys, bowels and skin. It expels toxins and rejuvenates the mental, glandular, hormonal and nervous systems. Alkaline juices are the best. The juices that are particularly recommended are carrot, beetroot and celery. For conditions such as ulcers cabbage juice is recommended. These fasts should only be taken when the body is strong and able to deal with the toxins that will be eliminated throughout the process.

All fasts should follow a programme of preparation, fasting and re-introduction to normal food consumption. Never start or finish a fast without taking these three necessary vital steps.

Overweight
After a certain age we are more prone to weight gain. It is around the age of 18 that this process begins, especially for meat-eaters. This is the age that we start to retain water.

Raw Vegetables
If you go on a raw vegetable diet, it does not matter what age you are, you will lose weight. Vegetables such as cucumbers, red and white radishes, celery and cabbage are the best ones to choose.

One Green Vegetable
A good weight-loss diet is to eat the same green vegetable for 30 days. This diet is also very good for cleansing the body and is very helpful in meditation. Make sure you break this diet with a single day of lemon juice, water and honey.

Reducing Drink
The following drink is good for losing weight and making it possible to work for 20 hours per day. Mix 225 ml (8 fl oz) of orange juice, two tablespoons of protein powder, two tablespoons of rice bran syrup, two tablespoons of chlorophyll, and one banana. You can live on this drink four times a day and eat nothing else. If you are strong and youthful, take three drinks per day and you will lose weight, be healthy and be taking care of yourself.

Royal Pickle

Mix the following ingredients in the following ratio: 0.45 kg (1 lb) peanut oil, 0.45 kg (1 lb) almond oil, 0.45 kg (1 lb) sesame oil, 113 g (¼ lb) olive oil, 1.50 kg (3¼ lb) of vinegar (white or malt, not chemical). Put it all in a jar then soak it in some chopped onions, ginger and garlic with a reasonable amount of black pepper. You can add some sea salt or a few red chillies if you want to make it hot. For every 0.90 kg (2 lb) of the mixture add 226 g (½ lb) of fennel seeds, 113 g (¼ lb) of cardamom seeds, 56 g (⅛ lb) of cinnamon, 28 g (1/16 lb) of cloves. Let it soak until the vinegar turns the ginger a reddish colour. When it is ready, eat two spoonfuls with your meals, and watch what happens.

Rice

Rice is not fattening, because it contains a little carbohydrate, which is essential for the brain, and it is necessary to promote the kidneys to secrete every toxin from the body. A diet of basmati rice with lemon juice and turmeric will let you lose weight and leave you feeling healthy and glowing.

Youthfulness

Cucumber Juice

If you are showing the signs of old age, eat cucumbers and take cucumber juice first thing in the morning.

Date Milk

Date milk is a very nourishing, energy-giving and youth-maintaining beverage.

Flax Seed Pudding

Flax seed pudding is made in exactly the same way as rice pudding, but is far more nutritious. It stimulates the entire metabolism and brings balance to all the metals in the body. It washes away any harmful toxins in the digestive tract, leaving you a picture of youth.

Olive oil and Milk
50 ml (1 fl oz) of olive oil with 225 ml (8 fl oz) of milk in the morning will keep you on good form.

Rosehips
Rosehips are a very good rejuvenating herb, it providing vitamin C, which is essential to the health of the body protein, collagen. For this reason rosehips keep the skin beautiful, youthful, prevent wrinkles, flabbiness and discoloration. They also keep the skin tight and smooth. Use cream with rosehips for the best results.

Sesame Oil and Milk
Drink 25 g (1 fl oz) of sesame oil with 175 ml (6 fl oz) of milk. This drink will keep you lively, fresh and young for the rest of your life.

Whey
Whey helps with digestion and elimination. It also helps prevent the harmful bacteria from forming by providing the proper nutrients for the beneficial bacteria in the intestinal tract. Whey also prevents constipation and is particularly high in the vitamin B2. A recipe for rejuvenation would be to take 5 g (4 oz) of vitamin C and 325 ml (12 fl oz) of whey. Make sure that the whey originates from curds and whey. Powdered and tablet forms are not as effective. Take this drink three times a day.

Liver

Foods that benefit the liver are artichokes, beetroot, carrots, celery juice, mangoes, onions and red radishes. The artichoke is known as medicine for the liver. This food rejuvenates this vital organ. Beetroot in any form cleanses the liver. 40 days of beetroot, carrots and onions with a layer of cheese melted on the top will have an excellent cleansing effect on the liver. Drink a mixture of carrot and beetroot juice. Yogi Bhajan has recommended that the juice is 25% beetroot juice and the rest carrot. This drink will greatly benefit the liver.

When the liver is unhealthy, the very best thing you can do is take watermelon juice, salt, yogurt, and a thin drink of Japanese Daiken radish. First thing in the morning take the radish juice. If your urine becomes reddish in colour, heed the warning that something is wrong. Begin to eat a very protective diet. Every three months, for one week, cleansing the liver is a must and diet is the only way. Live on yogurt for a week, but it must be fresh. When you use salt you must use black pepper as well, and when you use honey you must use lemons, too. This period will also help the spleen. During this week sweating exercise would be very helpful.

Prevention of liver problems

It is essential to avoid the following things in life to ensure proper functioning of the liver: heavy, half-cooked foods; foods that take hours to digest; greasy foods; meat; eggs; chemicals and animal fat; .all forms of alcohol and any stimulant drink that speeds up the digestion. If you have to eat after sunset, avoid eating within two hours of retiring for the night. Try to keep the stomach half-empty and do not drink while you are eating. Food should be light and easily digested. The liver becomes overtaxed if meals are closer than four hours apart. Also nibbling all day long is bad for the liver.

Diet for Women

It is particularly important for women not to eat after sunset or to have heavy meals at any time. The heaviest meal should be at lunchtime, never dinner. Try to make dinner as light and as digestible as possible.

Acids and Cholesterol

Alcoholic drinks and smoking are not good for women, in particular. Nor are coffee and other heavy stimulants. In addition, eggs, which are cholesterol-producing, are more dangerous for women than for men. The best diet is raw food. Women need proportionally more citrus, plums, peaches, papayas, raisins and dates. All types of seeds are a must because these foods are eliminated fast. Other recommended foods are green chillies, watermelon, beetroot, and all green vegetables.

A Vegetable Meal

It is strongly recommended that women have one meal of steamed vegetables every day, otherwise constant nibbling will lead to weight gain.

Curry

There is an ancient sutra that claims that this curry will prevent you from looking a day over 18. Take onions, garlic, ginger, garbanzo flour, lemon juice, and turmeric and add to yoghurt or buttermilk. Place on the heat and begin to stir. Then add almonds and other nuts, apricot kernels, walnuts, zucchini, watermelon and pumpkin seeds, green chillies and lemons. Almonds are for the eyes, watermelon seeds for anaemia, and walnuts for the brain. Turmeric is the most healing root for the body and for purifying the blood. It keeps a person beautiful.

Fruits

The following fruits are excellent for women: peaches, plums, papayas, figs, pears, guava, bananas, pomegranates, mangoes and orange juice. Green chillies are a must for women, helping to prevent waste pockets developing in the intestinal tract.

Salt and Sugar

Women should avoid salt and use lemons instead. Salt and sugar is her biggest enemy, as they take away her biggest weapon, her beauty. If you eat sugar, it must be raw, such as ghur.

Green Chillies

There is a scripture that states that women can live without men, but not without green chillies. Green chillies prevent mouth odour, constipation, giving the richest source of vitamin C and the most needed thing for women, chlorophyll.

Turmeric

Turmeric is the friendliest substance for women's internal organs so try adding it to as many meals as possible. Use it during cooking, rather than adding it afterwards.

Wheat Berries

Women should fast one day a week on just wheat berries for the intestinal tract, skin and beauty. Steamed wheat berries are the most sacred thing for the skin. They will make your skin shine like gold, enhance your sense of taste, build strong gums and teeth, prevent intestinal problems and strengthen your lower back. You can take boiled wheat berries, with honey and milk.

Diet for Men

There are certain diets that are a must for men.

Tri-Root, Saffron and Nuts

For substance, endurance, nerves and potent semen there is a potency food made of ginger, onion, garlic, saffron, pistachio nuts and almonds. Steam the onion, ginger and garlic in the ratio of 3:2:1 by weight, saffron ⅛ the amount of the ginger, a maximum of 50 pistachios and no more than 40 almonds. Blend this with a little honey and eat on toast. Remember, the onion, garlic and ginger are the trinity roots, the trident of life. The yogis recommended that this food be eaten only once a week. The day you take it should be a day of physical exercise, as you want the food to be digested and then sweated out through the skin.

Aubergine

In the ancient tradition, aubergine was called 'the testicles of God'. This is another food that enhances potency and vitality.

Golden Fruits

Figs can turn men into highly sexual and creative beings. Take between 20 and 25 figs, blend them with yogurt and drink the mixture. The figs need to be fresh not dried. The mixture should be thick so that you eat it with a spoon. You can go for a week to ten days on this. In the scriptures it says that if there is any sexual or nervous disability, this can correct it. For a normal healthy person, you should go on this diet for a week.

Garlic

Garlic gives sexual energy, which can be channelled into creativity. Men should eat two cloves of garlic a day. You can take it in a capsule, rather than raw, if you wish. But the male system requires it.

Nutmeg

Nutmeg lowers high blood pressure and it immediately brings temporary impotency. Such are the powerful effects of the little nut. For men who cannot control their sexual behaviour and ejaculation, this little nut will be Divine for them.

Courgettes

For all imbalances and misuse of your body, you should go on a fast, and should you decide to do a really good one, then just eat raw courgette for two weeks. Eat as much as you like. Start on the New Moon and go on until the Full Moon. Decide when the courgette is in season and begin. Eat the little, raw, young ones, when the skin is very tender.

Recipes

Mung Bean Salad and Rice

1 cup mung beans (soak overnight)
1 cup basmati rice
9 cups of water
4–6 cups of chopped assorted vegetables (carrots, celery, courgette, broccoli, etc.)
2 chopped onions
⅓ cup minced ginger root
8–10 cloves of garlic
1 heaped teaspoon of turmeric
½ teaspoon of pepper
1 heaped teaspoon of garam masala
1 teaspoon of crushed red chillies
1 tablespoon of sweet basil
2 bay leaves
seeds of 5 cardamom pods
salt or tamari sauce to taste

Wash the beans and rice. Bring the water to the boil, add the mung beans and let them boil over a medium-high flame. The mung beans will take three times longer to cook than the rice and vegetables. The mung beans need to be cooked until they begin to split. Bring another pan of water to the boil and then add the rice. Cook the rice normally and then add to the mung beans. Prepare the vegetables. Add the vegetables to the beans and the rice. Heat oil (½ cup) in large frying pan. Add onions, ginger and garlic and sauté over medium-high flame until they begin to brown. Add the spices but not the salt or herbs. When well done, combine the onions with the cooking beans and rice. You will now need to stir the dish quite often, to prevent scorching. Add herbs. Continue to cook, until well done over a medium-low flame. The consistency should be rich, thick and soup-like. Serve with yogurt or with cheese on top. This dish is pre-digested and is excellent for the sick, the elderly or for young children.

Yogi Tea

Start with 300 g (10 oz) per cup and brew at least 4 cups at once. For each cup you will need:

> 3 cloves
> 4 green cardamom pods
> 4 peppercorns
> ½ stick of cinnamon
> 1 slice of ginger root

Boil 10–15 minutes. Then add ¼ teaspoon of black tea. After 2 minutes add ½ cup of milk per cup of liquid. Heat to the boiling point and remove immediately. Strain and add honey to taste.

Golden Milk

> ⅛ teaspoon turmeric
> 3 cardamom pods
> ¼ cup of water

Simmer 5–7 minutes, then add 1 cup milk.
Bring to the boil point, but do not boil.
Add 2 tablespoons almond oil (cold-pressed).
Make sure the almond oil is added after the heating of the milk.

You can add honey or maple syrup to taste. Drink warm.

Vitamin and Mineral Sources

Vitamin A
Apples, bananas, carrots, papayas, white strings inside bananas and oranges

Vitamin B
Apples, coconut, papayas

Vitamin C
Apples, carrots, coconut milk, grapes, green chillies, lemons, olives (extremely high), oranges, papayas, rosehips

Calcium
Apples, bananas, cabbage, carrots, dairy products, figs, lemons, oranges, papayas, parsley, sesame seeds, watercress

Chlorine
Coconut, pineapple, watercress

Vitamin D
Papayas

Vitamin E
Sunflower seeds

Fluorine
Horseradish

Iodine
Coconut

Iron
Apples, apricots, bananas, parsley

Lecithin
Sesame seeds

Magnesium
Apples, coconut, grapes, lemons, oranges, sesame seeds

Mineral salts
Coconut milk

Phosphorus
Bananas (very high), coconut, olive, red chillies

Potassium
Apples, bananas, coconut, grapes, horseradish, lemons, olives (best), oranges, parsley, sesame seeds, courgettes

Protein
Apples, coconut (has all amino acids and is a complete protein)

Sodium
Apples, bananas, oranges

Sulphur
Chilli peppers, garlic, horseradish, onions, parsley, watercress

Zinc
Sunflower seeds

Beauty

This section is mainly for women, as it contains yogic advice on beauty and how to achieve balance. The main things to remember:

○ Eat nurturing food
○ Take cold showers to flush the capillaries
○ Sweat 15 minutes per day so that the glands can secrete
○ Wait 4 hours after eating before going to bed
○ Try to keep your food seasonal
○ Massage your skin daily with almond oil

First thing in the morning, take a cold shower. It will open your capillaries and bring the blood to the surface of the skin, leaving you with vitalized and youthful skin. With the opening of the capillaries, the inner organs get flushed of any toxins that built up while you were sleeping.

It is especially important for women to get the cold water on their breasts and to massage them under the shower. This extra attention to the breast area is much-needed since there is a rise in breast cancer in the Western world.

When you wake up, get out of bed slowly. To jump out as soon as you open your eyes is damaging to the nervous system and will throw your aura out for the rest of the day. It is much better to do some stretches in bed and stimulate your whole body before you get up.

Another important piece of advice for women is to sit on your heels in Rock Pose after eating. This is the very best position to aid your digestion; ideally you should sit like this for seven minutes after eating. If you do this every day, you will hardly ever become ill.

The yogis had a special method for washing their hair. They would massage it with oil and yogurt and a fragrance of their liking. Massage the hair thoroughly and then wrap it in a towel. Keep it wrapped for a couple of hours before shampooing. Let your hair dry naturally. It is very important that you get your hair, scalp and skull exposed to the sun once a week.

For Rejuvenation of Your Entire System
Fill a jar with rose petals that have not been touched by hands. Pour honey over them and let it sit for a year. Then eat the honey.

For Red or Sore Eyes
Place grated raw potatoes between two slices of muslin or gauze. Apply to the eyes while resting. Replace the potatoes with fresh ones when they have dried out. Relax.

To Keep a Person Beautiful
Take turmeric. It is very healing and purifying to the body. It is especially good for women.

For Clear Skin
The best inner cosmetic is camomile.

For Depression
If you eat a banana first thing in the morning and at 4.00pm, along with a handful of raisins, you will never become depressed. The banana gives you potassium. With your daily levels maintained you are unlikely to suffer.

To Maintain Health
Women should drink three cups of yogi tea per day.

Three-Day Cleanse
Three days of eating only watermelon will completely cleanse your body. Men should allow 11 days.

To Reduce the Ageing Process
The more pears a woman eats, the younger she will look. Pears make up for iron deficiency in the blood.

To Increase Sexual Energy
Eat aubergine at least once a week. It will give you sexual energy. It is full of iron and when it is cooked correctly it is one of the most cleansing foods you can have.

For Digestion
Broccoli has the most digestible protein for women.

For Skin and Scalp
Rosemary is very good for the skin and scalp.

Weight Loss
Alfalfa tea is great for weight loss.

Menstrual Cramp
Dong Quai is known as 'women's ginseng' (also known as Tang Kuei). It is especially helpful for menstrual cramps and hypertension.

For Morning Sickness
To relieve morning sickness and to relax the cervix during childbirth, drink red raspberry leaf tea.

For the Skin
Massage the skin daily with almond oil, for softness and tone.

Sources and Resources

Please contact the author direct at:
siridatta@anaharta.com
www.anaharta.com for retreats, workshops,
classes and Siri Datta's updates

Or write to me at:
Michael Alcock Management
96 Farringdon Road
London. EC1R 3EA
UK.

If you are looking for a Kundalini Yoga
teacher in your area, you can find a listing
of certified Kundalini Yoga teachers
worldwide at the internet site:
www.kundaliniyoga.com

IKTYA (International Kundalini Yoga Teachers' Association)
Contact Person: Nam Kaur Khalsa,
Executive Director
Route 2, Box 4 Shady Lane,
Espanola, NM 87532
Phone: 505-753-0423 FAX: 505-753-5982
Website: www.yogibhajan.com
Organization of Kundalini Yoga Teachers.

Membership includes a listing in the
Annual Teacher's Directory, discounts on
selected yoga products, and subscription
to *Kundalini Rising* a newsletter for Teachers.
It provides a listing of Teachers worldwide.

3H0 Events
Route 2, Box 132-D, Espanola,
New Mexico 87532
Toll Free: 888-346-2420, 505-753-6341,
ext. 121 / FAX: 505-753-1999

For information on Winter and Summer
Solstice gatherings, White Tantric Yoga
schedules around the US, Europe, Mexico,
and Canada, special events, and camps.
For a list of various activities throughout
the year related to the 3HO Foundation,
which sponsors events related to Kundalini
Yoga and organizes gatherings worldwide,
visit the following website:
www.3ho.org
3HO International Headquarters
PO Box 351149
Los Angeles, CA 90035

Yogi Bhajan Home Page
www.yogibhajan.com

Many books, tapes and videos related to
Kundalini Yoga can be purchased via:
Ancient Healing Ways.
Call for a free catalogue
Route 3, Box 259,
Espanola, NM 87532
Toll Free: 800-359-2940
505-747-2860 / FAX: 505-747-2868
Supplier of books, audio and videotapes,
herbal formulas, healing teas, and body-
care products formulated by Yogi Bhajan.

Magazines and Newsletters

Science of Keeping Up
Published by the 3HO Foundation. Write
or email 3HO to be put on the mailing list.

Kundalini Rising
Official newsletter of the International
Kundalini Yoga Teachers Association.
IKYTA
3HO International Headquarters
New Mexico Office
Route 2, Box 4
Shady Lane
Espanola, NM 87532

Aquarian Times
Available through Ancient Healing Ways

About the Author

I was born in Newbury, Berkshire, 22 December 1969 and as I was an only child, I was showered with rather a lot of love and attention. From an early age I became aware of my growing feelings of compassion for others. My instincts told me how to comfort others by showing them their light and, in turn, this eased their pain. Throughout my life I have always had an understanding of the bigger picture, an inner knowing of an intelligent source, which we all came from.

After school I went to art college and then studied fashion design at Middlesex University. In 1996 I set up my own fashion business, an instant hit in Japan. Later, in 1997, I experienced a much deeper insight into the spiritual world. It was at this point that I stumbled across Kundalini Yoga.

Within minutes into my first class tears were rolling down my cheeks, many emotions were released, one after the other. I had found what I had been looking for. This form of yoga opened up the connection to my soul at a much deeper level. The transformation was so quick; I had literally become alive. I became focused, strong and healthy. People remarked how I oozed vitality and happiness, even though I was going through one of the most difficult periods in my life.

I decided that this sacred technology had to be shared with humankind, so in 1998 I began the teacher-training course with SKY (School of Kundalini Yoga). After completing the course I began teaching, before and after my working day. But my life became a struggle. There was a constant knowing that I had to leave the fashion industry and dedicate my life to teaching others how to free themselves. After two years, I finally decided to teach full time and dedicate myself to living in full truth, and motivating others to do the same.

The opportunities came thick and fast. The day I told my business partner that I was resigning was the day I received my spiritual name from Yogi Bhajan. Siri Datta translates as 'the great giver'.

I began teaching at private health clubs, hotels, alternative health practices, my home, festivals and yoga spaces. My classes embodied a huge rush of transformation and excitement and became wild and unpredictable.

In 2001, there were many more changes to come. After completing Reiki I, II and Masters I met another beloved teacher, Anrul Ullah, who humbly reconnected me with the Christ Consciousness that resides in us all within the chamber of the heart.

What is the goal now?
As it's always been, to inspire and uplift humanity, while living life as true to the source as can be.

One way I have been doing this is by holding retreats. These are not quiet, meditative and peaceful spaces; they are full of the wonder of life. Sunrise at Stonehenge, sunset at Glastonbury Tor, climbing trees, leaf catching, staying up for the whole of the duration of the retreat (if you want to) and endless tears and laughter.

I will write many more books, not just on yoga, but words of inspiration and elevation that will resonate with many people. There is a growing movement within humanity, and I have decided to become a beacon for the truth. I also plan to release a range of yoga videos to accompany the books.

My philosophy is 'A glimpse of your Self will change your life in that moment. It is my intention to be one of the brightest mirrors that you have ever looked into'.

Glossary

3HO foundation.	Healthy, Happy, Holy Organisation
Adi Shakti	Primal Power
Ajna	Brow Chakra
Akashic Records	An energetic record of everything that has ever taken place, all thoughts, actions and deeds
Ambrosial Hours	Between 4 – 7am
Anahata	Heart Chakra
Apana	Elimination, the eliminating force, the out-going
Asana	Yogic posture
Astral Body	The energetic body that transmits information to and from the astral field
Astral Field	The realm of thoughts, emotions and feelings
Atma	Soul
Aura	Energetic field that surrounds the body
Ayurveda	Ancient Hindu holistic medical system
Bhagavad Gita	Ancient Hindu scripture written in 2,500 BC, means Lord's Song
Bhakti	Devotion
Bhandh	Lock
Bij Mantra	Seed sound
Breath of Fire	Rapid nasal breath that cleanses and revitalises
Brow Point	The area between the eyebrows
Caduceus	Ancient symbol now used for the modern-day medical industry
Cannon fire breath	Powerful exhalation either through nose or mouth
Chakras	Energy centres
Dharana	Concentration
Dharma	Righteousness
Dhyana	Meditation

Ego	The false Self. The Personality, the perceived self
Electromagnetic field	Aura
Elements	Earth, air, fire, water and ether
Endocrine	Glandular system
Enlightenment	A fully realized being, full state of awareness
Ether	Space
Gheranda	Tantric sage
Gheranda Samhita	Ancient text on Tantra
God	Generator, organizer, destroyer (deliverer). God is a 'word'.
Golden Chain	The sacred link between the great spiritual teachers and yogic masters of all times and the teacher or practitioner of Kundalini Yoga
Gurbani	Sacred language of the Sikhs.
Guru	'Gu' means darkness, 'ru' means light. The giver of technology, the teacher, the process from darkness to light
Guru Nanak	First Sikh Guru
Guru Ram Das	The fourth guru of the Sikhs, patron saint of Kundalini Yoga
Gyan	Knowledge
Harbhajan Singh Puri	Birth name of Yogi Bhajan
Hatha Yoga	Yogic path primarily using postures, and development of the will
Hatha Yoga Pradipika	Classic source of Hatha Yoga practice
Ida	Left nerve channel, relates to left nostril and the energy of the Moon
Ini	Endearment
Jalandhara Bhandh	Neck Lock
Jugit	Union
Karma	Action and reaction. The cosmic law of cause and effect
Karta Purkh	The working God
King Janaka	Early Raj Yogi
Kirlian Photography	Photography that records energetic fields around physical objects
KRI	Kundalini Research Institute
Kriya	Specific combination of yogic postures; literally 'a completed action'

Knot of Brahman	Energetic knot at the Base Chakra
Knot of Shiva	Energetic knot at the Brow Chakra
Knot of Vishnu	Energetic knot at the Heart Centre
Kundalini	The nerve of the soul; literally 'the curl in the hair of the beloved'
Maha Bandh	The Great Lock
Mahan Tantric	Master of white tantric yoga; currently Yogi Bhajan
Manipura	The Navel Centre, Third Chakra
Mantra	Sound current that controls mental vibration. Words of power; mental vibration to the infinite mind.
Meridians	Energy pathways in the body
Mudra	Yogic hand position
Mul Bandh	The Root Lock
Muladhara	The first of the chakras, the Root/Base Chakra
Naad	The universal code behind human communication
Nadis	Psychic nerve channels
Niyamas	Rules of personal conduct
Ojas	Cerebro-spinal fluid
Paramatma	The Universal soul
Pineal	A small gland in the head, connected to the Crown Chakra
Pingala	Right nerve channel, relates to right nostril; Sun energy
Pituitary	The master gland
Prana	The energy of the atom, essence of life, the inhalation, life force
Pranayama	Yogic breathing technique
Pratyahara	Control of the senses
Psyche	Energetic blueprint
Raj	Royal
Rig Veda	Ancient scripture known as 'Knowledge of praise', 5,000 BC
Sadhana	Spiritual daily practice
Sage	A person in tune with the Universe, a 'knower' of the unseen worlds
Sahasrara	The Crown Chakra, Seventh Chakra
Samadhi	Enlightenment
Sant Hazara Singh	Spiral teacher of Yogi Bhajan and the Mahan Tantric

Sanskrit	One of the first documented languages
Shabd	Sound; sound current
Shakti	Woman; the feminine aspect of God
Shiva	A Hindu god, known as the 'destroyer'
Shiva Langham	That which is surrounded
Siddhasana	Perfect Pose – a sitting posture
Siddis	The 'magical' powers attained through yoga
Sikh	Seeker of Truth
Siri Datta	The great giver
Sitali Pranayama	A cleansing breath that cools the body
Sivananda yoga	A form of yoga from Sri Swami Sivananda
Sukhasana	Yogic posture known as Easy Pose
Sushmana	Central spinal channel
Sutra	Text
Svadisthana	The Second Chakra
Takhat	The 'High Throne'
Tantra	Union of the two polarities, male and female
Tapa	Physic Heat
Tattva	Element
Uddiyana	The Diaphragm Lock
Vedas	Ancient Hindu Scriptures
Vishnu	A Hindu god, known as the 'sustainer'
Vishuddhi	The Throat Chakra, Fifth Chakra
Whistle breath	An inhale or exhale through the mouth making a whistle sound
Yamas	Universal ethical principles
Yoga	Union, the science of uniting individual consciousness with universal consciousness
Yoga Sutras	The text by Patanjali that documents the full practice of yoga
Yogi	One who has attained a state of yoga
Yogi Bhajan	Master of Kundalini Yoga and current Mahan Tantric of White Tantric Yoga

Bibliography

Yoga for Health and Healing, from the teachings of Yogi Bhajan, compiled by Alice B. Clagett and Elandra Kirsten Meredith (Bookpeople, 1995)

Kundalini Yoga: Guidelines for Sadhana, from the teachings of Yogi Bhajan

Self Experience, Harijot Kaur Khalsa

Self Knowledge, Harijot Kaur Khalsa

The Inner Workout Manual, KRI

Physical Wisdom, Harijot Kaur Khalsa

Survival Kit, Yogi Bhajan, compiled by Elandra Kirsten Meredith and Alice B. Clagett

Owners Manual for the Human Body, Editor: Harijot Kaur Khalsa (KRI, 1997)

The New Book of Yoga, The Sivananda Yoga Centre (Ebury Press, 2000)

Kundalini Yoga: The flow of Eternal Power, Shakti Parwha Kaur Khalsa (The Penguin Group, 1998)

The Chakras, Naomi Ozaniec (Headway, 1999)

Hatha Yoga, Godfrey Devereux (Thorsons, 2001)

The Ancient Art of Self-Healing, Yogi Bhajan

Patanjali Yoga Sutras, Swami Prabhavananda

Index

Make
www.thorsonselement.com
your online sanctuary

Get online information, inspiration and guidance to help you on the path to physical and spiritual well-being. Drawing on the integrity and vision of our authors and titles, and with health advice, articles, astrology, tarot, a meditation zone, author interviews and events listings, www.thorsonselement.com is a great alternative to help create space and peace in our lives.

So if you've always wondered about practising yoga, following an allergy-free diet, using the tarot or getting a life coach, we can point you in the right direction.

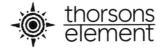

thorsons
element